AF477244

Regulatory Aspects of Pharmaceutical Quality System
Brief Introduction

Regulatory Aspects of Pharmaceutical Quality System
Brief Introduction

Prof. (Dr.) Arun Kumar Pandey

PhD. M.Pharm

Sr. Vice President - R & D

Dr. Pavan Kumar Rawat

PhD, M.Pharm

Mr. Shantanu D. Shinde

M.Pharm, PGDM

**Alkem Laboratories Limited,
Mumbai**

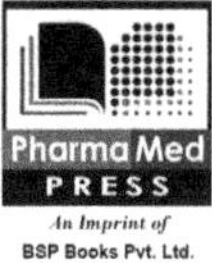

PharmaMed Press

An imprint of BSP Books pvt. Ltd

4-4-309/316, Giriraj Lane,
Sultan Bazar, Hyderabad - 500 095.

Regulatory Aspects of Pharmaceutical Quality System – Brief Introduction
by Prof. (Dr.) Arun Kumar Pandey

© 2024, *by Publisher*

Disclaimer: The authors and the publishers have taken due care to provide the authentic, reliable and up to date information related to the subject. However, neither the authors nor the publisher shall be responsible for any liability for any damage caused as a result of use of this book. The respective user must check the accuracy from other sources too.

Published by:

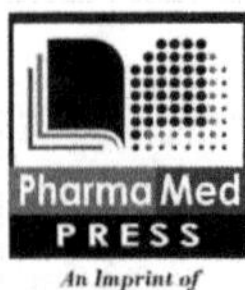

PharmaMed Press
An imprint of BSP Books Pvt. Ltd.
4-4-309/316, Giriraj Lane, Sultan Bazar, Hyderabad - 500 095.
Phone: 040-23445688; Fax: 91+40-23445611
e-mail: info@pharmamedpress.com
www.pharmamedpress.com/pharmamedpress.net

ISBN: 978-81-961468-5-6 (Hardback)

Preface

This book is designed as a textbook for teaching basic principles of quality assurance and the relevant guidelines for B. Pharm and M. Pharm students.

Although there are numerous books on the science of quality assurance these books cover different areas of the discipline in varying depths and provide limited insight into contemporary practices and practical applications.

Each of these textbooks, by itself, does not provide an integrated approach to the students. This leads the students as well as the teachers to refer to many textbooks to develop an overall understanding of the basic guidelines related to quality. In an attempt to overcome these challenges, this book provides a unified perspective of the overall field to the students as well as instructors.

The students need to know the basic industry guidelines, the application of these principles to the design of quality management, and the relevance of these principles to the fundamental aspects of drugs. Another important aspect of teaching that is urgently needed in our pharmacy students. curricula are to expose students to the latest developments in the Industry.

Exposure of students to these latest developments is critical to the successful training of future pharmacists, because these therapeutic modalities and options are likely to be significant in the future.

All these principles and applications need to be integrated within a single textbook, so that the student develops a better overall understanding of the principles involved in the effective designing of guidelines and be aware that how quality plays an important role in the overall well-being of the community and finally our country.

This book covers an in-depth discussion of how guidelines can be used for the design, development, and evaluation of various dosage form You have an updated, contemporary, new book that can serve as a textbook for Pharma students and a valuable resource for the novice in the pharmaceutic field.

- Author

Contents

Introduction

The quality in the pharmaceutical industry has become a very important topic. Since the world has gathered together to harmonize its practices and guides and the launching of the FDA current good manufacturing practices – the cGMP; for the 21st century – there has been a growing awareness for the significance of the quality of the pharmaceutical products (Woodcock, 2004).

This awareness is represented through the appearance of several definitions defining exactly what the quality of the medicine should be (LEE and Webb, 2009). Many articles were written to demonstrate the special nature of the product-customer relationship of medicine and patients (Woodcock, 2004).

Also the important role of governments was emphasized through the joint statement between the International Pharmaceutical Federation; IPF; and the International Federation of Pharmaceutical Manufacturers Associations; IFPMA; to ensure the safety of medicinal products in order to protect the patient (FIP Council, 1999), providing that the pharmaceutical industry is one of the most closely regulated industries for more than 50 years (Woodcock, 2004). Since 2002, FDA began an initiative to address cGMP for the 21st century (Woodcock, 2004). This effort involved taking new looks at both the regulatory and industrial systems for insuring drug quality (Larson, 2006).

As agency guidance is increasingly aligned with the principles of these founding fathers of modern-day quality, it is worth exploring Juran's and Deming's views on leadership and learning how they evolved from engineers to philosophers in management.

After World War II, Juran and Deming both traveled to Japan to help rebuild the country's economy. Their efforts helped revolutionize the quality system of Japan and started a quality revolution that the rest of the world could not help but notice. Evidence of Juran and Deming's work is present today in FDA guidance documents and regulations, as well as in other industries that have quality system regulations.

Leaders in the pharmaceutical industry must recognize that as quality systems have evolved, so too have the expectations and responsibilities they must fulfill. Quality cannot be an afterthought with any product, nor can it be the responsibility of any one department. Quality must be instilled within an organization and designed into processes and systems. Most importantly, perhaps, the culture of quality must begin with the leaders in the organization. These concepts are also detailed within the "Q10 Pharmaceutical Quality System" Guidance for Industry.

Every government allocates a substantial proportion of its total health budget to medicines. This proportion tends to be greatest in developing countries, where it may exceed 40%.

Without assurance that these medicines are relevant to priority health needs and that they meet acceptable standards of quality, safety and efficacy, any health service is evidently compromised. In developing countries considerable administrative and technical effort is directed to ensuring that patients receive effective medicines of good quality. It is crucial to the objective of health for all that a reliable system of medicines control be brought within the reach of every country.

The supply of essential medicines of good quality was identified as one of the prerequisites for the delivery of health care at the International Conference on Primary Health Care in Alma-Ata in 1978. Similarly, the Conference of Experts on the Rational Use of Drugs, held in Nairobi in 1985, and WHO's Revised Drug Strategy, adopted by the World Health Assembly in May 1986, identified the effective functioning of national drug regulation and control systems as the only means to assure safety and quality of medicines.

Yet the World Health Assembly continues to express great concern about the quality, safety and efficacy of medicines, particularly those products or active pharmaceutical substances imported into, or produced in, developing countries. In recent years counterfeit products have infiltrated certain markets in disquieting proportions.

Since the founding of WHO, the World Health Assembly has adopted many resolutions requesting the Organization to develop international standards, recommendations and instruments to assure the quality of medicines, whether produced and traded nationally or internationally.

Both for manufacturers and at national level, GMP are an important part of a comprehensive system of quality assurance. They also represent the technical standard upon which the WHO Certification Scheme on the Quality of Pharmaceutical Products Moving in International Commerce is based.

In many markets, quality competition is at least as important as price competition and this trend is bound to continue. With the prospects of more stringent product liability legislation and the threat of heavy financial penalties for products and services which fail to meet safety, good manufacturing compliance (GMP) or functional requirements, profitable trading will depend on sound Quality Assurance best practices. Material resources are becoming scarce and most expensive, and it is therefore economically desirable to minimize losses on scrap products by more effective quality control.

Quality has been defined as the totality of features and characteristics of a product or service that bears on its ability to satisfy a given need; and Quality Assurance as all activities and functions concerned with the attainment of quality. The concepts include sound marketing analysis to establish customers' requirements and satisfactions; ensuring that designs reflect these requirements in fitness for purpose at an economic cost, reliability considerations and the practical constraints imposed by manufacturing capability; organizing and controlling production to consistently conform to design specifications; and following up these actions with adequate after sales services and the feedback of relevant field data.

This importance of reliable product quality cannot be over emphasized when one is attempting to break into new markets and win new business. It is now an established fact that many pharmaceutical potential markets are far more demanding in this respect than were customers in the past. In addition, more legislation and regulations relating to product conformance and reliability are coming into operation. It is recognized that the most effective advertisement for a product or service is the satisfied customer. Making a conquest sale has been estimated to cost a company ten times the repeat sale. The performance of the product is totally dependent on good design and development coupled with conformance during manufacture to the specification and build process.

The quality of a product does not occur by accident. People throughout an organization do not always carry out instructions, or perform their role correctly. It is the continuing task of quality management to deal with this situation and ensure that all members of the industrial team are aware of their quality responsibilities and are accountable for their actions. Quality must be designed into products – discipline, attitude and inventiveness must be encouraged to create easy to make and easy to use fool proof products. Quality must then be planned into manufacture – methods must be devised so that the easiest way to do the job is the right one; so that, where appropriate, worker interest is created; and elsewhere complete control is built into the process. Finally, quality must be built into the product – the people concerned with the cutting, fitting and assembling must be well trained and enthusiastically led to achieve "right first time" production. This is the simple overall formula, but it is by no means simple to put into practice.

To make quality assurance an effective part of business, Senior Management must be clearly committed to developing and implementing an effective Quality Policy. The implementation of such a policy involves everyone in the company. It must be clearly recognized that every employee (from board to shop floor) is responsible for ensuring that GMP and good quality practices are achieved. All departments within a company must be held accountable within their own spheres of influence for ensuring that for the selling price of the product, the required quality standards are inherent within the design and methods, processes specified and the materials and equipment provided.

The Quality Executive

The role of Quality Executive in industry is now-a-days highly specialized. The post is not one that can normally be used as a "stepping stone" in a promotional ladder. The reason is fairly obvious; a person in a Quality Executive role can gain popularity and short term achievement by effecting cost reductions and in making favorable decisions, etc., only for the company to have to pay later. There are good reasons as to why there are dangers in making short term assessments on achievements in this sphere. It is a job that is essentially involved in long term consequences and as a consequence it is not always a particularly popular job.

The idea that the work of quality organizations was simply that of "inspecting out" defective work which had already been produced was widespread in the past, particularly in management circles. As a corollary, it also followed that the kind of person required was low level and fairly non-technical. In this belief, management has not kept abreast of the developments which began during the 1939/1945 world war and which have been accelerating in the last decade.

It is true to say, particularly over the last decade, that there has been considerable technical advance in the nature of the work of quality specialists. These have taken them a long way away from the old idea of inspection pure and simple. Today's emphasis in the work of quality specialist is towards the prevention of defect altogether. The modern view is that "no inspection is good inspection". In order to achieve this goal, a high degree of professionalism is required in these new techniques, which call for considerable study and practical experiences leading to qualification as quality practitioners.

In addition to these recognizable technical factors, an urgent need has arisen for quality professionals to broaden their experience into a field which, until now, would have been considered to be completely foreign. This need has developed due to the imminence of international and national legislation relating to product liability. This has taken the quality professional into the fields of insurance and the law. It has also meant, although most of these other disciplines do not yet appear to realize the fact, a great widening of the circle of operations in a company to which the quality professional must direct his attention for assurance purposes. The scope of this new, wider area and the urgency which must be attached to it are such that it is clear that the Quality Assurance function will have to be applied throughout a company organization.

Quality cannot however be achieved solely by the Quality Executive, it depends on everyone being actively involved. The Quality Executive's contribution is essentially one of coordinating the efforts of others to ensure the achievement of quality by communicating information on the many aspects affecting quality to all concerned and exercising control over quality monitoring throughout the organization. It must be the task/goal of all managers to ensure that the quality function of their own departments is fulfilled. This places a heavy responsibility on all senior managers.

The recent years have seen an explosive increase in the information and progress in various sub disciplines of pharmaceutical sciences as well as the basic sciences, which forms the foundation of this applied science. This date book incorporates both the basics of quality assurance emphasizing on importance of quality and the regulatory guidelines that are currently followed by India as well as foreign agencies and the changes currently underway in a balanced fashion to enable a holistic development of the next generation of students. I am confident that this book will enable a deeper understanding of fundamental principles and a wider perspective related to quality and its practice to our next generation of students.

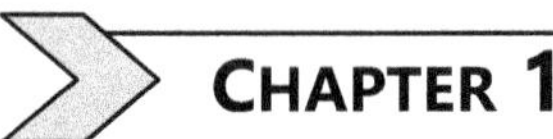

CHAPTER 1

Introduction to Quality Management System

A Quality Management System (QMS) is defined as a set of interrelated or interacting elements such as policies, objectives, Aim, procedures, processes, and resources that are established individually or collectively to guide an organization.

Management Responsibility: Senior management is responsible for assigning a management representative to develop and maintain the QMS, acting as representative in all issues concerning quality. Conflicts of interest should be avoided, and the management representative shall be given sufficient authority. The necessary resources shall be available to the management representative, and the responsibilities placed on any one individual shall not be so extensive as to present any risk to product quality. Senior management should ensure:

➢ The QMS takes into account all applicable guidelines and regulations.

➢ Management reviews are performed on a regular basis.

➢ The quality manual, quality policies, and quality objectives are all in place.

➢ Job descriptions, responsibilities, and authorities are clearly understood within the organization.

The Top Ten Responsibilities of the Pharmaceutical Quality Unit are as follows,

➢ To establish the quality system

➢ To ensure quality system is audit compliant

➢ To establish procedures and specifications

➢ To establish manufacturing controls

➢ To perform laboratory tests or examinations

➢ To review and approve or reject all things cGMP

➢ To ensure investigation of non-conformance

➢ To keep management informed

➢ To describe responsibilities in writing

➢ To remain independent

Elements of Quality Management System

A quality management system typically consists of four facets

Quality Planning: Process of translating quality policy into processes, procedures, and instructions to achieve measurable objectives and requirements

Quality Assurance: Planned and methodical activities executed as part of a quality system to provide confidence that process, product, or service requirements for quality are being satisfied

Quality Control: Act of monitoring, appraising, and correcting a process, product, or service to ensure requirements for quality are being satisfied

Quality Improvement: Process of analyzing performance and taking methodical, systemic actions to improve it

Quality Management System Planning: The organization should take into account applicable regulatory requirements, the size of the company, the complexity of materials and products, and other critical activities when developing the QMS structure.

The QMS should be designed to maintain its robustness, even when changes occur. The quality policy, quality objectives, and quality risk management are essential in developing a QMS and should be defined by senior management.

An appropriate QMS should include, but is not limited to an organizational structure capable of supporting the elements of the quality policy and quality objectives.

➢ Written policies, procedures, records, and agreements that can demonstrate how materials, products, and services will meet established quality specifications

➢ Qualification monitoring and review of outsourced activities

➢ Competence development of personnel through training and promoting awareness of individual job impact on quality

➢ Deviations and complaints handling

➢ Continuous improvement through corrective action and preventative action (CAPA), audits, and management reviews, and QMS planning and commitment

Communication: The organization should establish communication channels that ensure the timely flow of information within the organization and to supply chain partners. Customers should be notified of any changes in packaging, handling, storage, transportation, or documentation (e.g., material safety data sheets or labels).

Communication within the supply chain should be coordinated to determine proper timing of transported and received products, taking into account holiday schedules, weekends, and other interruptions.

Documentation: The organization should have in place a system to control documents and data that are part of the QMS. Since documentation is an essential element of any QMS, having written instructions regarding processes and evidence that activities were completed is essential.

The written instructions should be well-structured and clear in order to facilitate understanding and compliance. Electronic documentation should meet the requirements stated under the Control of documents section and the electronic document control system should be validated.

Control of Documents: The goal is to ensure that all documents in use are updated, approved in a timely manner, and that the current version is in use. These practices prevent obsolete or non -approved documents from being used, which could lead to error. The organization should have a written procedure for controlling documents and establishing formal control regarding identification, revision, approval, distribution, and withdrawal of obsolete copies.

All documents should be approved and training should be performed prior to their use. All documents that relate to product quality and the QMS should be reviewed on a regular basis. The management representative, or a properly qualified designee, should approve these documents. Controlled documents should include a unique identifier, date of issue and revision, and the parties responsible for preparing, approving, and revising the documents.

Employees should have free and timely access to all quality documents that impact their work. The documents should be written in straightforward language that allows full understanding. Documents should be retained for a period required by national and international regulatory bodies (see Control of Records).

At least one obsolete copy should be retained for history after the first revision. External documents such as pharmacopeias, ISO standards, and regulatory acts and guidelines should also be controlled within the QMS.

Quality Manual

The organization should prepare a quality manual or equivalent documentation, such as a site master file, describing at least:

➤ Brief information on the organization (name, contact information) and its relation to other companies

➤ Activities as licensed by the competent authorities, if applicable

➤ Types of materials, products, and services handled

➤ Scope of the QMS

➤ Overview of the QMS showing the constitutive elements of the system and the structure of documentation used

➤ Quality policy

- Quality objectives
- Identification of the processes and their sequences, linkages, and interdependences
- Organizational chart
- Matrix of key personnel responsibilities
- Reference to supporting procedures and documents, such as a validation master plan

List of Standard Operating Procedures (SOPs)

Senior management should establish, authorize, and communicate a quality policy. The policy should be suitable for the organization and describe the overall intentions of the organization regarding quality.

The quality policy should be subject to periodic management review in order to maintain its appropriateness. Personnel within the organization should understand the quality policy and how their work affects it.

- Responsibilities
- Brief description of the processes to be validated
- Equipment, facilities, vehicles, and utilities to be commissioned and qualified and to what extent [installation qualification (IQ), operation qualification (OQ), and performance qualification (PQ)]
- Templates for the protocols and reports
- Requalification and revalidation triggers change control

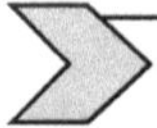 **Standard Operating Procedures (SOPs)**

Written procedures should ensure that materials and products are held in accordance with their labeling instructions and associated regulatory requirements. The written procedures should provide all the steps needed to complete a process and ensure consistency and standard outcomes.

Organizations should establish written procedures for all processes within the organization relating to product or material handling and the QMS, including but not limited to:

- How the material or product is stored, and the controls necessary to ensure the appropriateness of the storage conditions.
- How and when a material or product should be moved from one transport container or vehicle to another.
- How materials and products are handled when equipment malfunctions or when there are delays in distribution due to customs holds, weather, etc.
- How to communicate to necessary supply chain partners.

Product Specification and Material Safety Data Sheet (MSDS)

The organization should have written specifications for incoming materials and outgoing finished materials or products. Specifications can be used for procuring, selling, and quality control analysis. An MSDS should be prepared according to national or international requirements and should be provided with the shipment for transportation, importation, or export.

Protocols

Protocols are applicable for commissioning, qualification, and validation studies. The management representative or an authorized designee should approve them.

Schedules

Organizations should have approved schedules for preventive maintenance, calibration, training, and requalification or revalidation studies.

Forms

Forms required for the operation of the QMS and the provision of the material, product, or service should be part of the document control system.

Labels

Labels are fundamental to material identification. For this reason, any label change should be communicated to down-stream supply chain partners. Label-generating systems and processes should be secure, controlled, documented, and validated.

Suitable verification records should be maintained and each container should be appropriately identified and labeled. Labels applied, even to small containers, should be clear, indelible, unambiguous, and permanently fixed in the format established by the manufacturer, packager, or re-packager.

The label should include wording or icons to emphasize storage and transportation conditions, handling requirements, and hazards. The use of symbols that are recognized by international organizations is strongly recommended.

Labeling

In the context of GDP, labeling is not limited to manufacturing information but may also include shipping and exporting information added to product tertiary packaging.

Control of Records

Records are special kinds of documents that provide evidence of activities performed. For this reason, they should be legible, clear, indelible, identifiable, traceable, and established immediately after performing an activity. The organization should have a written procedure for the control of records

These procedures should establish ways for identifying, storing, and protecting records, in order to avoid deterioration and damage. Electronic records and automated data-capture systems should meet the requirements for the control of records and should be validated. Records should be signed and dated by the person who performed the activity. Corrections to entries should be signed and dated, leaving the original entry legible with an explanation for the change, if applicable, especially if this may not be obvious to subsequent reviewers. Examples of records include: shipment receipts, invoices, packing or repacking batch records, temperature and relative humidity monitoring logs, etc.

Records should be retained for purchases and sales. They should show the date of purchase or supply, the material, product identification (name, batch or serial number, if applicable), product amount, the name and address of the supplier or consignee, and the name and address of the carrier

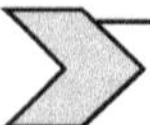 ## Resources of Firm Management

Senior management should provide appropriate resources (personnel, facilities, equipment, material, and time) to implement and remain in compliance with GDPs.

1. Personnel Responsibilities and Authorities

The organization should have an organizational chart showing the organizational structure. There should be an appropriate number of personnel to avoid excessive duties being placed on one individual, which can compromise quality. Third parties may be contracted, but they should be audited for competency in executing the duties for which they are to be contracted.

The organization should establish job descriptions, with clearly defined responsibilities and authorities, that are clearly understood by personnel. Personnel should not be subjected to conflicts of interest that can adversely affect the quality of products within the supply chain.

2. Training

The organization should establish written procedures for training. These procedures should describe at least the following: who can be a trainer, competencies of a trainer, how training needs are identified, types of training practices (e.g., self-instructional, classes, on-the-job training, web-based training), and how training effectiveness will be evaluated.

Initial and ongoing training should be given based on an approved training schedule. Training needs should be identified and linked to job description, complexity of duties and types of material handled (e.g., narcotics, radiopharmaceuticals), management reviews, and any kind of human resources program for competence development.

Basic training on GDP should be given to all employees, with the goal of developing awareness outside of related job functions. Records of all training should be kept, and effectiveness of training should be assessed.

3. Hygiene, Occupational Health, and Safety

Written procedures related to hygiene and apparel should be provided, and their use should be enforced. Appropriate apparel should be provided to personnel in order to avoid contamination of both product and personnel.

The organization should be responsible for apparel cleaning. Personal protective equipment should be provided and training in its use given. Any source of product contamination or occupational hazard should be prohibited, including but not limited to: jewelry, food, medicines, or tobacco products.

These can be sources of contamination and occupational hazards, and they should be prohibited in product storage and handling areas.

Premises and Equipment Premises should be designed to maintain the quality and integrity of the materials and products stored.

Buildings should be constructed in such a way that they are appropriate for the intended operations, taking into account:

- Security and safety
- Product characteristics
- Ease of cleaning and maintenance
- Logical flow of personnel and material
- Means of preventing mix-ups and cross-contamination
- Ergonomic measures
- Any local, national, or international requirements
- Necessary environmental controls
- Facilities should be of adequate size for their intended use to prevent overcrowding. Storage should be orderly and provide segregation of quarantined, approved, rejected, returned, recalled, and adulterated products.

Receiving, sampling, and shipping areas should be segregated. Facilities should protect products and materials from inclement weather as necessary. Products with special-handling authorization, such as narcotics, should be segregated and locked in a secure area. Radiopharmaceuticals and radiolabeled materials should be contained in dedicated locked storage areas.

Products with fire or explosion risks should also be kept in dedicated areas specially constructed for this purpose. Products that require special storage conditions with regard to temperature and humidity should also be segregated.

Restrooms, lunchrooms, and social amenities for employees should be separated from the storage and shipping areas. Smoking, eating, and drinking should not be allowed in any storage or shipping area. Access control systems should be in place to prevent unauthorized access to storage areas.

Alarm systems should also be in place. Adequate precautions should be taken to prevent theft and diversion of products. Facilities should have controls and contingency plans to mitigate risks of fire, water, explosion, and terrorism.

Written procedures should be established for cleaning, sanitation, pest control, receiving, storing, and shipping activities. Cleaning and sanitation procedures should indicate the frequency of cleaning as well as the materials and methods used.

Pest control procedures should ensure the prevention of contamination as well as the safe use of pesticides. Records should be kept. All equipment and monitoring devices used to hold and move products within the supply chain should be appropriate for their intended use. Written procedures on how to operate the equipment should be established and approved.

Organizations should establish written procedures for calibration, repair, and preventive maintenance, taking into account at least the following:

➢ Responsibilities of the in-house staff and third parties, if applicable

➢ Calibration and maintenance agreements

➢ Change control, requalification, or recalibration needs

➢ Calibration and preventive maintenance schedules

➢ Spare parts, equipment, and monitoring device management Actions to be taken if equipment or monitoring devices are found out of specification prior to recalibration

➢ Protections against damage during handling, calibration, and maintenance

Forms for recording calibration, repair, and preventive maintenance activities:

If any change is made to the equipment after repair, the organization should evaluate whether a requalification or recalibration is necessary. Calibration should be performed against traceable standards (national or international) and according to an approved schedule.

Monitoring devices should be safeguarded from actions that can invalidate the calibration. Risk assessment should be used to determine the frequency of calibration.

Commissioning and qualification should also be completed. The extent of these efforts should be determined in the validation master plan. Work Environment Organizations should ensure that appropriate work environments and conditions are provided for the products to be handled and for the personnel handling them.

A written procedure should be established by the organization determining the requirements for cleanliness, luminosity, temperature, relative humidity, pest control, personal garments, and health. Any contaminated or potentially contaminated product (e.g., complaint samples, returns, used medical devices sent for repair) should be carefully handled to avoid contamination of other products and personnel.

Material

All material handled within the supply chain or used to ensure the quality and integrity along the supply chain (e.g., reagents, growth media, transport vehicles, lubricants, HVAC spare parts) should have a written specification, which should be used for purchasing, selling, and quality control, where applicable.

A written procedure for identification and storage of all material should be in place. Quality control analysis for incoming materials should be performed (e.g., imported materials and products). Written procedures should be in place for sampling, analysis, and disposition of the products, and records kept. Quality control laboratories, where applicable, should be constructed for this purpose and based on national or international requirements. Written procedures should be established for handling controlled drug substances and drug products prior to, during, and after analysis. Obsolete materials should be destroyed according to written procedures and documented.

Transport Vehicles

All vehicles used in supply chain activities, such as semitrailer trucks, vans, trucks, tanker trucks, trains, airplanes, sea vessels, mail delivery vehicles, motorcycles, emergency medical services, and industry representatives' automobiles, should be suitable for their intended purpose. They can be considered in-transit storage and require the precautions needed to maintain product quality and integrity.

Dedicated temperature-controlled transport vehicles should be qualified. For other vehicles, shipment monitoring is required as appropriate to demonstrate the protection of the drug product or material of any storage area.

Organizations owning or leasing their transportation vehicles should have a written plan for the purchase, maintenance, and replacement of vehicles used to transport products. They should also have a transport vehicle log listing at least: vehicle identification, chassis, age, condition, mileage, operational status, and insurance policy number, if applicable.

Vehicle cleaning procedures should be written and records kept. Preventive maintenance and pest control should be done according to approved schedules, and written procedures and records kept.

Cleaning validation should be performed if the product is in contact with the transportation vehicle (e.g., tanker trucks for excipients). If there are problems with vehicles during the transportation process (e.g., breakdowns, accidents, loss of fuel), cargo should be protected against environmental factors, thefts, and diversions, and a nonconformance report should be opened. Such provisions should be included in the service level agreement.

Operations

Procurement Organizations should establish written procedures for procurement, taking into account at least:

- Purchase based on material and product specification
- Supplier qualification
- Responsibilities
- Purchase approvals
- Purchase forms and records

All intended activities and services should also comply with all local laws and regulations. The organization should establish a written procedure for how suppliers are selected and evaluated, and the criteria for qualification.

Supplier qualification audits should be handled as established in the Audits section. Records should be kept. A list of all qualified suppliers should be in place. Shipping and Receiving Organizations should establish a written procedure for receiving goods and determining the appropriate checks for this process.

A checklist can be utilized as a reminder of what to inspect and what to record, taking into account: purchase order, material or product name, amount ordered, amount received, batches or serial numbers received, expiry date, manufacturer name, marketing authorization holder name, carrier name, date and hour of receiving, cargo conditions, appearance, and whether the supplier or carrier is licensed to handle the material or product. If computerized systems are used to control orders, materials, products in stock, supplier and customer files, and carriers, the organization should record material or product item codes and internal lot numbers, if applicable.

Where appropriate, the transport vehicle should be inspected before unloading to verify that adequate protection from contamination was maintained during transit. Deliveries should be verified at receipt in order to check that containers were not damaged and that the consignment corresponds to the order.

Appropriate delivery records (e.g., transport vehicle movement documents, receiving and delivery records, data logging records, temperature records and similar devices, bills of lading, house air waybills, master air waybills) should be reviewed by each receiving organization in the supply chain to determine if the product has been subjected to any transportation delays or other events that could have exposed the product to undesirable conditions.

Each supply chain partner should ensure that its respective service level agreements and supporting documents cover delivery and receiving responsibilities of the transactional parties. All incoming materials and products should be quarantined. After disposition is confirmed, products should be transferred to their respective storage areas, according to their classification and storage specification. When products arrive at warehouse loading docks and other arrival areas, they should be transferred as quickly as possible to a designated storage area within a time period that is consistent with the risk assessment in place.

Sampling

Sampling should be performed if analytical control is required on incoming materials. The organization should establish a written procedure for sampling, including at least: sample identification, quantity, protection and safety procedures for the sample and remaining product, method for communicating results, and changes in product status and location.

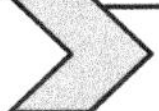

Storage

Organizations should establish a written procedure for material and product storage. Each material and product should have a storage specification regarding temperature, relative humidity, and other special requirements (e.g., controlled substances and drug products and radiopharmaceuticals).

No material or product should be stored directly on the floor. Pallets should be used to hold material and products and should not cause contamination. If wood pallets or packages are used, they should comply with international requirements (e.g., International Standards for Phytosanitary Measures).

Storage areas should be qualified and a temperature mapping and monitoring program should be in place (see 1083.2). Organizations should establish a written procedure for inventory control, which should be checked periodically. If any inventory deviation is found, a nonconformance report should be opened and the appropriate authorities informed, if applicable (e.g., controlled products and radiopharmaceuticals).

Products beyond their expiry date should be removed from the saleable stock and assigned "rejected" status while awaiting destruction (see 1083.2). Sales Organizations should establish a written procedure for sale and customer qualification. This is applicable only for business-to-business partners, Regulatory authorizations for all intended activities or services (e.g., wholesale, transport) are mandatory except brokering. Copies of authorizations should be requested periodically to ensure that the "qualified" status is maintained. Lists of qualified suppliers and customers should be maintained.

Product Selection and Packaging

A written procedure should be established by the organization ensuring that the correct product was selected, properly packaged, and dispatched. Products should be selected on a first-expired, first-out basis.

Appropriate packages should be in place ensuring that the product will be preserved throughout storage and distribution. Package qualification tests should be performed according to approved protocols.

Transportation Products and materials should be transported in such a way that any specified conditions are maintained and nothing impacts the quality and integrity of the product or material.

A written procedure should be established by the organization, including at least:

- Responsibilities

- Approvals for subcontracting

- Methods for defining transportation routes

- Capacities and limitations of transportation systems, loading patterns (e.g., first- out, last-in), and insurance needs.

Carriers should record, at least: product name, amount, batches or serial numbers, sender name, recipient name, carrier route, receiving and delivery date and hour, duration and condition of transport, vehicle identification, mileage, and operator name. Transportation vehicles should be qualified and maintained. Transportation should be planned in a way that promotes a rational use of resources (e.g., transportation vehicles, fuels) and provides better logistics to avoid delays and product stress. Only licensed drivers, pilots, and operators can conduct transportation vehicles. All national and international (if applicable) regulations should be followed. A global positioning system (GPS) should be used to aid delivery and to track the transportation vehicle

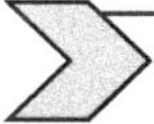

Outsourcing Activities

A written agreement should be developed and signed for all outsourced activities related to the procurement of materials and services. The suitability and competence of the parties to carry out their responsibilities should be investigated.

All duties, information, and responsibilities required for both the service supplier and the customer should be clearly described. Audits should be performed to assess the appropriateness of the contractor.

Subcontractors may be used but only with formal agreements among all parties, such as the service supplier, customer, and the subcontractor. Organizations should establish written procedures to regulate any prospective outsourced activities and the related agreements.

The performance of contractors should be monitored on a regular basis, and improvements should be identified and implemented.

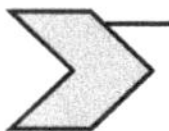

Complaints, Deviations, Returns, Recalls, Counterfeits, and Reprocess and Rework Products

Complaints

A written procedure for complaint handling should be in place, including at least:

Instructions for receiving complaints and communication channels available to the complainant

Complaint log

Complaint investigation form with basic information about the complainant (e.g., name, address, country, contact person, phone number, e-mail), the product or service complaint (e.g., product name, batch number, expiry date, detailed description of complaint, amount of product with alleged problem, order number, carrier name and route, shipping and storage conditions, date of complaint), results of investigation, and conclusion (confirmed, non-confirmed, or adulterated product). Each complaint investigation form should have a unique identification number.

- Instructions for recommending CAPA.
- The criteria for choosing appropriate CAPA depends on the nature and the frequency of the complaint.

- Description of how customer complaints are addressed and resolved, and which types of complaint warrant notification of regulatory authorities.
- Monthly reports and trend analyses, including times for complaint handling.
- A complaint officer with comprehensive knowledge of the supply chain should be assigned since this person will be responsible for choosing the most applicable investigation approach.
- The complaint officer also acts as a link among other areas within the organization, such as marketing, operations, quality, maintenance, regulatory, and legal affairs. Legal affairs should be notified if a suspicious or counterfeit product is identified or a breach of contract is suspected.
- Records should be kept for each complaint. Monthly reports should be compiled in order to allow the evaluation of the number and the nature of complaints received. A trend analysis of complaints should be performed and used as input for management review.

Deviations

A written procedure for handling deviations should be in place. If any deviation occurs, a nonconformance report should be opened and a unique identification number assigned. The investigation should include at least the following:

- Complete description of the deviation
- Where, when, and how the deviation was found
- Actions taken to prevent non authorized use of the nonconforming product or nonconforming service
- Frequency of deviation
- Description of how the deviation impacts quality
- Necessity to trigger a corrective action
- The management representative should approve all decisions concerning products or services with deviations. Records should be kept.

Returns

A written procedure for handling returns should be in place. A return form should be opened for each product that is sent back to the organization. A risk-based evaluation should be performed to determine if the product will be accepted for restocking and resale or if it will be destroyed.

Restocking should be accepted only once, with the exception of medical devices. During the evaluation, returned products should be kept in a segregated area specifically for returns until final disposition.

Each return form should have a unique identification number. The evaluation should take into account at least the following:

- Reasons for return
- Appearance and integrity of the original packaging
- Evidence of conditions in which the cargo was transported and stored throughout the entire time
- Duration of time between the original shipment and its return
- Authenticity of the product
- Representative sampling for quality control analysis
- Expiry date and batch number
- Information from any track-and-trace system in place

The QMS management representative should approve all decisions concerning returns prior to disposition of the returned goods (e.g., restocking or destruction). Records should be kept, and the product should be labeled according to its returned status.

The organization should inform customers if there is a returned product included in their order, prior to shipment.

Recalls

All supply chain partners are responsible for the quality and integrity of products under their control. Any time a deviation is found that affects the integrity of a marketed material or product, a recall should be promptly initiated.

The organization should have a written procedure establishing the steps for recalling products, including at least:

- Responsibilities for the recall operation
- Instructions for tracking the delivery information on recalled products
- Recall communications, such as customer letters and their approval
- Frequency of recall inventory queries and regulatory updates
- Necessary documentation (e.g., distribution records with names, addresses, phone or fax numbers, contact persons, e-mail addresses, batch or serial numbers, quantities)
- Identification and segregation of recalled products
- Time frames for recall
- Forms for recording the recall progress and the final report
- Any other national or international regulatory requirements

The QMS management representative is responsible for the entire recall process applicable to the organization, including the communication within the organization and with other supply chain partners, regulatory authorities, and certification bodies. Regulatory and legal affairs departments should be aware of the recalling progress. Recalled products should be kept segregated and labeled with their recalled status. Disposition of recalled products should be recorded. Effectiveness assessment of the recall procedure should be done periodically.

Adulterated Materials and Products

The organization should have a written procedure for handling and notifying authorities if an adulterated or suspected adulterated material or product is identified within the supply chain. The marketing authorization holder or the manufacturer, if different, should also be notified.

Adulterated materials and products should be kept segregated and labeled with their adulterated status. Disposition of these products should be recorded and records kept.

Counterfeit Products

The term "counterfeit drug" means "a drug which, or the container or labeling of which, without authorization, bears the trademark, trade name, or other identifying mark, imprint, or device, or any likeness thereof, of a drug manufacturer, processor, packer, or distributor other than the person or persons who in fact manufactured, processed, packed, or distributed such drug and which thereby falsely purports or is represented to be the product of, or to have been packed or distributed by, such other drug manufacturer, processor, packer, or distributor" [21 U.S.C. §321(g)(2) (2004)]. This is comparable to the term "falsified medicinal product" used in the EU.

Reprocess and Rework Products

Organizations should have a written procedure for handling reprocess and rework products. A change control should be opened prior to rework and records kept. [NOTE— This item applies to packagers and repackagers.]

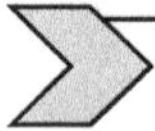

Monitoring and Improvements

Product or Service Quality Reviews (PSQR)

Product quality reviews are required of manufacturers. However, service providers are also responsible for product quality while the product is within their control. For this reason, a product or service quality review should be done by distributors, freight providers, importers, and exporters.

PSQRs should be performed at least annually, and summary reports on each material, product, or transportation route should be available for regulatory inspections, audits, and management reviews.

A written SOP should have at least the following, as applicable:

- Period of the review

- Product name and dosage form

- Batch numbers and quantities per batch handled

- Carrier routes

- Deviations or complaints found per product, batch, and carrier route

Audits

Audits are a valuable tool for evaluating QMS effectiveness, along with regulatory inspections. It is necessary to verify if a supply chain partner complies with QMS planning and with GDP requirements.

Internal audits are conducted by or on behalf of the organization itself. External audits are performed by, or on behalf of, organizations that might have an interest in partnering with another organization (e.g., customer for supplier qualification).

The audit criteria, scope, and objective should be clearly defined. Auditors should not be subjected to conflicts of interest that may adversely affect the audit, and for this reason auditors should not audit their own work. The organization should have a written SOP establishing the rationale for audits, which should include at least the following:

- Responsibilities for the audit program

- Description of who can be an auditor

- Competencies of an auditor

- Auditor training

- Frequency of audits

- Instructions for planning an audit (e.g., audit feasibility, criteria, scope, objective, expected duration, auditor team, travel arrangements, translators, necessary clothes and protective equipment, matters related to confidentiality)

- Instructions for conducting on-site audit activities (e.g., opening and closing meetings; collecting and verifying information methods, such as interviews, document reviews, observation activities)

- Audit reports and follow-up

- Audits should be performed at least once a year according to a schedule and discussed during management reviews.

Management Reviews

The QMS should be reviewed periodically (e.g., in each quarter of the year) in order to assess problems, trends, corrections, preventions, regulatory updates, and concerns. Inputs for the management reviews should include but are not limited to:

- Previous management review reports
- Audit and regulatory inspection reports and actions in place
- Complaints, nonconformance, returns, and recalls
- Detected or potential counterfeiting
- Status and effectiveness of the CAPA system
- New or updated regulatory requirements
- Quality policy
- Quality objectives metrics as key performance indicators
- Change control reports
- Quality manual

The outputs of the management reviews are:

- Recommendations for improvement of the system, processes, products, or services
- Demand for resources Corrective Action and Preventive Action (CAPA) Organizations should have a written SOP establishing the provisions for corrective and preventive actions as well as instructions for how they should be handled within the organization. Root cause analysis should be performed to identify the cause of a critical deviation in order to implement corrective action. The use of quality tools for this investigation (e.g., Ishikawa diagram) is recommended.
- Confirmed complaints, critical deviations, and audits can trigger an investigation. Trend analyses, frequent non confirmed complaints, and audits can trigger a preventive action. The effectiveness of the corrective or preventive action should be evaluated.
- Continuous Improvement Organizations should implement a systematic approach for performing QMS improvements. Management reviews, audits, regulatory inspections, and QMS planning initiatives are potential triggers for continuous improvement activities and should be followed up by senior management.

Validation

Validation efforts should be established in the validation master plan and should be based on risk assessment. Commissioning and Qualification

Commissioning (site acceptance test or factory acceptance test), installation qualification (IQ), operation qualification (OQ), and performance qualification (PQ) should be performed to provide written documentation that equipment, warehouse facilities, and vehicles are installed correctly, operate as expected, and perform as required to ensure product and service quality.

Qualification and validation studies should be performed after instruments are calibrated. As appropriate, commissioning includes, but is not limited to, air-handling units, water systems, boilers, chillers, generators and emergency power systems, access control and alarm systems, safety and security systems, and repackaging equipment.

Commissioning efforts do not differentiate between occupational risk and risk to the product. Commissioning documents and reports can be incorporated into the qualification as part of IQ and OQ efforts.

After commissioning and qualification, periodic tests should be performed in order to ensure that utilities, equipment, and systems are working properly.

Any modification should be done according to change control procedures, and records should be kept. Analytical methods, cleaning validation, and process validation analytical methods used to perform the quality control of products, especially for imported products, should be verified or validated according to approved protocol (see Validation of Compendial Procedures 1225, Verification of Compendial Procedures 1226, and national or international requirements).

Cleaning validation should be performed on equipment and utensils if any packaging or repackaging operation exposes them to the product. Process validation should also be done for all critical operations that have the potential to compromise the quality and integrity of the product or service.

Challenges to the process should simulate regular storage and transportation conditions as well as out-of-specification conditions. Performance qualification can substitute for process validation. After validation, any modification should be done according to change control procedures, and records should be kept.

Computerized Systems

Computerized systems should be validated according to approved protocols prior to their use. Systems already in place should also be validated. The extent of validation depends on the risk to or impact of the software on product or service quality. Validation is not applied to software that has no impact on quality. An inventory of computerized systems should be done periodically, including at least:

* Software identification (name, version)
* Software supplier

- Processes where software is used
- Process owner
- Risk assessment
- Status (validated, not validated, validation in progress, not applicable)

A multidisciplinary team with representatives from information technology, quality, and operations should be responsible for protocols and report approvals. Responsibilities for the tests should be assigned in the protocols.

Software validation tests should cover

Security (e.g., access levels, profiles, responsibilities inclusion, exclusion, or changing profiles)

- Data validity (e.g., challenge the software with entries above and below specification and with entry value errors).
- Documentation (e.g., software design in accordance with user requirements and other documents)
- Functionality (e.g., calculations, operations). [NOTE-Most of the functionality tests for embedded software are covered during equipment qualification (installation, operation, and performance qualifications).]
- Data integrity (e.g., changes, traceability, backup, recovery, protection) After validation, any modification to the system should be done according to change control procedures. Records should be kept.

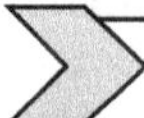 **Change Control**

Improvements, management reviews, complaints and deviation handling, and other monitoring systems can trigger change. The organization should have a written procedure describing the steps for change control.

It should include: responsibilities, an impact assessment of the change based on risk, necessary validation, documentation review, regulatory impact, and the necessity to have planned activities for the change.

The organization should have a team of experts to evaluate the change, including representatives from operations, quality, regulatory and legal affairs, and logistics and maintenance.

The QMS management representative should approve all changes prior to implementation. An effectiveness assessment should be carried out to confirm that QMS integrity after implementation has not changed.

Customers and regulatory bodies should be notified of any MSDS changes in packaging, handling, storage, transportation, or documentation (e.g., MSDS or labels).

Regulatory Affairs

Supply chain partners should apply for all required licenses and authorizations for their activities. These documents should be readily available for regulatory inspections and supplier and customer audits upon request.

This also applies to subcontractors. Only drug products holding marketing authorizations can be distributed within the commercial supply chain, except for investigational drug products.

A written procedure for this kind of product should be established by the organization, determining all precautions needed to ensure integrity through the supply chain. A written procedure for controlled drug substances, drug products, and radiopharmaceuticals inventory should be in place, and records should be available for audit by competent authorities. Senior management should assign a person to be in charge of all regulatory updates, applications, and issues regarding storage and distribution of materials and products handled within the organization. This person should also work to increase the regulatory awareness within the organization.

Quality Management System in Testing Laboratories

Professionals of testing laboratories have shown increasing interest in understanding the QMS and attaining accreditation status for their services since the introduction of international standards for the quality management system (QMS).

Thus Quality assurance therefore is defined as the process or the end of the process which confirms for the integrity of a product to meet the standard for the intended use. Quality assurance is an obligation automatically imposed on the manufacturer of any product to ensure that it meets the needs of the end-user in the measures intended for use. For the end-user, the benchmark of quality is perfection they cannot allow less than 100%.

Elements of the Quality Management System

The laboratory is a complex system, involving many steps of activity and many people. The complexity of the system requires that many processes and procedures be performed properly. Therefore, the QMS model, which looks at the entire system, is very important for achieving good laboratory performance. The QMS is defined as a 'management system to direct and control an organization with regard to quality. The QMS covers the laboratory activities, including drug sampling, analysis and reporting. The QMS consists of documentation of the laboratory policy and objectives, system procedures and instructions for assuring the quality of its results to meet safety and regulatory requirements and to satisfy the needs of the customers.

Pharmaceutical Quality Management System

It is applicable to drug products, including biotechnology and biological products, throughout the product lifecycle the systems supporting the development and manufacture of pharmaceutical drug substances. It includes,

- Pharmaceutical Development
- Manufacturing and development of APIs.
- Manufacture of medical kits and devices for investigation.
- Development of medical delivery systems.
- Pilot plant scale-up activities
- Manufacturing process of formulation
- Development of medical devices for accurate dosing Analytical Method Development
- Acquisition and control of materials
- Provision of facilities, utilities, and equipment Production (including packaging and labelling) Quality control and assurance.
- Release
- Storage During Product Technology Transfer During product discontinuation
- Retention of sample and related documentation
- Continued product assessment and reporting

The term quality cannot be confined to one definition. It is tensile in nature and people define it in their own ways but one thing is common in all and that is satisfaction. Manufacturer is satisfied if the product meets it specification and consumer is happy when the particular product fulfils his need. Anyways, Quality is unavoidable thing today and one cannot ignore it. When it comes in context of Pharma then Quality is a legal issue and must be maintained in pharmaceutical products. The present chapter focuses on some aspects and need of maintaining Quality in Pharma through Quality Management System pharmaceutical products.

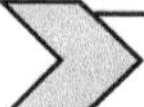 **Important Questions**

1. What are the goals of a quality management system?
2. What value does a quality management system add?
3. What are the Benefits of QMS?
4. What are the prerequisites for implementing and certifying a QMS?
5. How return and recalls an important part of quality management system?

6.   Change control is defined with target closure dates? Explain.

7.   What are the different elements of Pharmaceutical Quality management system?

8.   How important is CAPA once deviation is reported? Explain Briefly.

9.   What is the difference between deviation and change control?

10. What is the difference between CAPA and QMS?

11. Define and explain in brief advantages of Audit.

12. Define SOP and advantage of SOP.

CHAPTER 2

Good Manufacturing Practice Regulations - A Brief Scenario

GMP is that part of Quality Assurance which ensures that products are consistently produced and controlled to the quality standard appropriate to their intended use and as required by the marketing authorization.

Good Manufacturing Practices (GMPs): are regulations that describe the methods, equipment, facilities, and controls required for producing: Human and veterinary products Medical devices and Processed food.

Usually see "cGMP" – where c = current, to emphasize that the expectations are dynamic. It is designed to minimize the risks involved in any pharmaceutical production that cannot be eliminated through testing the final product.

These regulations, which have the force of law, require that manufacturers, processors, and packagers of drugs, medical devices, some food, and blood products take protective steps to ensure that their products are safe, pure, and effective.

Require a quality approach to manufacturing, enabling companies to minimize or eliminate instances of contamination, mix-ups, and errors.

Protects the consumer from purchasing a product, which is not effective or even dangerous. GMP regulations address issues including record keeping, personnel qualifications, sanitation, cleanliness, equipment verification, process validation, and complaint handling.

In short GMP makes the difference between nearly right and exactly right.

Why GMP?

Final testing of the product cannot ensure the quality, efficiency and safety.

- Final testing may always not detect contamination, error, etc. Conformance to the predetermined specification.
- To minimize contamination eg:- microbial contamination.
- To eliminate error.
- To produce product of consistent quality.

- Government requirement.
- Ensure quality product.
- Reduce rejects, recalls
- Satisfied customers.
- Company image and reputation.

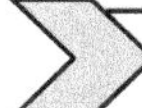 ## Code of Federal Regulations (CFR)

It is the Portion of FDA.

The collection of final regulations published in the federal register (daily published records of proposed rules, final rules, meeting notices, etc).

Divided into 50 titles, Current regulations of GMP appear in part 210 (title 21) of code of federal regulations published by USFDA.

Evolution of GMP

1963: - first GMP publication- USA

1971: -first revision

1978: - Major revision

Current regulation of GMP appear in part 210 (title 21) of code of federal regulations published by USFDA.

Main Risks Without GMP

Unexpected contamination of products, causing damage to health or even death Incorrect labels on containers, which could mean that patients receive the wrong medicine

Insufficient or too much active ingredient, resulting in ineffective treatment or adverse effects.

Principles of GMP

Design and construct the facilities and equipments properly

- Follow written procedures and Instructions
- Document work
- Validate work
- Monitor facilities and equipment
- Write step by step operating procedures and work on instructions
- Design, develop and demonstrate job competence

- Protect against contamination
- Control components and product related processes
- Conduct planned and periodic audits

Parts of GMP

Good Manufacturing Practices for Premises and Materials

1. General Requirements

1.1   Location and surroundings

The factory buildings for manufacturing of drugs shall be so situated or shall have such measures as:

To avoid risk of contamination from external environment.

Any factory, which produces obnoxious odors, fumes, dust, smoke, chemical or biological emissions.

1.2   Building and premises

The building should be designed in such a way that permits manufacturing operations in hygienic conditions.

Compatible with other manufacturing operations.

Adequately provided with working space.

To avoid risk of mix-ups.

To avoid contamination.

Designed to avoid entry of pests, birds, rodents etc.

Interior surface should be smooth and free from cracks.

The production and dispensing area shall be well lightened, ventilated, and may have proper air handling system.

Proper drainage system as specified for various categories of products.

The walls and floors of manufacturing area shall be free from cracks and open joints to permit easy and effective cleaning.

1.3 Water system

There shall be validated system for treatment of water to render it potable.

Potable water should be used to perform all the operations except cleaning and washing. The storage tanks shall be cleaned periodically and records maintained by the licensee.

1.4 Disposal of waste

The disposal of sewage and effluents shall be in conformity with the requirements of Environment Pollution Control Board.

All bio-medical waste shall be destroyed as per the provisions of Bio-Medical Waste Rules, 1996.

Record shall be maintained.

Provision shall be made for proper storage of waste materials.

2. Warehousing area

Adequate areas for proper warehousing of various categories of materials and products.

Designed and adapted to ensure good storage conditions.

Quarantine area shall be clearly demarcated and restricted to authorized persons.

Separate sampling area for active raw materials and excipients.

3. Production area

Designed to allow the production preferably in uni-flow and with logical sequence of operations. Separate manufacturing facilities shall be provided for the manufacturing of contamination causing and potent products such as;

- β-lactam, sex hormones and cyto-toxic substance.
- Service lines shall be Well designed and constructed, shall be identified by colours. Direction of flow shall be marked.

Products intended for use in clinical trials should be manufactured in accordance with the requirements of this guideline, and where required by national legislation, in licensed facilities. Manufacturing operations should be controlled as appropriate to the phase of development and scale of manufacture.

Where activities are outsourced to contract facilities and the product(s) to be manufactured or controlled are intended for use in clinical trials, the contract must then clearly state, inter alia, the responsibilities of each party, compliance with this guideline and WHO GMP 610. Close cooperation between the contracting parties is essential.

Manufacturing operations

As process validation may not always be complete during the development phase of products, provisional quality attributes, process parameters and in-process controls should be identified, based on risk management principles and experience with the products or analogous products.

The necessary processing instructions should be identified and may be adapted based on Working document and the experience gained in production. Where processes such as mixing have not been validated, additional quality control testing may be necessary. For sterile investigational products, the sterility assurance should be no less than for commercial products.

Packaging and labelling

The packaging and labelling of investigational products are likely to be more complex and more liable to errors (which are also harder to detect) when "blinded" labels are used than for commercial products. Supervisory procedures such as label reconciliation, line clearance, and other controls, including independent checks by quality unit personnel, should be intensified accordingly. The packaging must ensure that the investigational product remains in good condition during transport and storage. Any opening of, or tampering with, the outer packaging during transport should be readily discernible.

Blinding operations

In the preparation of "blinded" products, the blind should be maintained until it is required to allow for the identification of the "blinded" product. The label expiry date should be assigned to ensure that the 'blind' is not broken

A coding system should be introduced to permit the proper identification of "blinded" products. The code, together with the randomization list, must permit the proper identification of the product, including any necessary traceability to the codes and batch number of the product before the blinding operation. Controls should be applied to verify the similarity in appearance and other physical characteristics such as the odour of "blinded" investigational products. Maintenance of Working document blinding during the study should be ensured and verification of effectiveness of blinding should be performed and recorded.

4. Ancillary areas

Rest and refreshment rooms shall be separate from other areas. Facility for changing, storing clothes and for washing and toilet purpose shall be easily accessible and adequate. Areas for housing animals shall be isolated and maintained as prescribed in rule 150- C (3) of D & C Rules, 1945.

5. Quality control area

Quality control laboratories shall be independent of the production areas, separate areas shall be provided each for physico-chemical, biological, microbiological or radio –isotope analysis.

Adequate space shall be provided to avoid mix-ups and cross contamination.

The design of the laboratory shall take into account the suitability of construction materials and ventilation.

Separate air handling units and radioisotopes testing areas. The laboratory shall be provided with regular supply of water of appropriate quality for cleaning and testing purposes.

Quality control should cover, for example, the sampling and testing of materials and products. The analytical procedures should be suitable for their intended purpose, ensuring that materials and products are not released for use or supply until their quality has been judged to be compliant with the specifications.

Each batch of product should be tested in accordance with the specifications included in the Product Specification File and should meet its acceptance criteria.

Bulk product release should cover all relevant factors including production conditions, the results of in-process testing, a review of manufacturing documentation and compliance with the Product Specification File and the order. Finished product release should cover, in addition to the bulk product assessment, all relevant factors including packaging conditions, the results of in-process testing, a review of packaging documentation and compliance with the Product Specification File and the order.

Reference and retention (control) samples of each batch of product should be retained.

Samples should be retained in the primary container used for the study or in a suitable bulk container for at least two years after the termination or completion of the clinical trial.

Retention samples should be kept until the clinical report has been submitted to the regulatory authorities or at least two years after the termination or completion of the relevant clinical trial, whichever is longest. This is in order to enable the confirmation of product identity in the event of, and as part of an investigation into, inconsistent trial results.

The storage location of reference and retention samples should be defined in a technical agreement between the sponsor and manufacturer(s) and should allow for timely access by the competent authorities.

The release of a batch of an investigational product should only occur after the designated responsible person and sponsor, as required, have certified that the product meets the relevant requirements. These requirements include the assessment of, as appropriate:

- batch records, including control reports, in-process test reports, changes, deviations and release reports demonstrating compliance with the product specification file, the order, and randomization code

- production conditions
- The qualification status of facilities, validation status of processes and methods, as appropriate
- The examination of finished packs
- where relevant, the results of any analyses or tests performed after importation;
- Stability reports
- The source and verification of conditions of storage and shipment
- Audit reports concerning the quality system of the manufacturer, where applicable
- Documents certifying that the manufacturer is authorized to manufacture investigational medicinal products or comparators for export by the appropriate authorities in the country of export
- Where relevant, regulatory requirements for marketing authorization, GMP standards applicable and any official verification of GMP compliance

6. Personnel

The manufacture and testing shall be conducted under direct supervision of qualified technical staff.

Personnel for QA & QC shall be qualified and experienced.

No. of personnel employed shall be adequate and in direct proportion to the workload.

Personnel in production and QC lab. shall receive training appropriate to the duties & responsibility assigned to them.

7. Health, clothing and sanitation of workers

The personnel handling beta-lactum antibiotics shall be tested for penicillin sensitivity before employment and those handling sex hormones, cytotoxic substances and other potent drugs shall be periodically examined for adverse effect.

Prior to employment, all personnel shall undergo medical examination including eye examination, and shall be free from tuberculosis, skin and other communicable or contagious diseases.

- **Clothing:**

    Protection of operator and product, highly potent products or those of particular risk.

    Need for special protective clothing.

    Personnel should not move between areas producing different products.

    Garments need to be cleaned

- **Health examinations:**

On recruitment for direct operators, repeated on regular basis

- **Training:**

Check Induction training for new operators includes basic personal hygiene training. Written procedures - to wash hands before entering a manufacturing area.

- **Illness:**

Staff with illness or open lesions should not handle starting materials, intermediates or finished products.

8. Manufacturing operations & controls

All manufacturing operations shall be carried out under the supervision of technical staff approved by the Licensing Authority. Each critical step in the process relating to the selection, weighing and measuring of raw material addition during various stages shall be performed by trained personnel under the direct personal supervision of approved technical staff.

The contents of all vessels and containers used in manufacture and storage during the various manufacturing stages shall be conspicuously labeled with the name of the product, batch no., batch size and stage of manufacture. Each label should be initialed and dated by the authorized technical staff. Products not prepared under aseptic conditions are required to be free from pathogens like Salmonella, Escherichia coli, Pyocyanea etc.

Precautions against mix–up and cross-contamination:

The licensee shall prevent mix-up and cross- contamination of drug material and drug product (from environmental dust) by proper air-handling system, pressure differential, segregation, status labeling and cleaning. Proper records and Standard Operating Procedures thereof shall be maintained.

The licensee shall ensure processing of sensitive drugs like Beta-Lactum antibiotics, sex hormones and cycotoxic substances in segregated areas or isolated production areas within the building with independent air-handling unit and proper pressure differentials. The effective segregation of these areas shall be validated with adequate records of maintenance and services. To prevent mix-ups during production stages, material under- process shall be conspicuously labeled to demonstrate their status. All equipment used for production shall be labeled with their current status.

Packaging lines shall be independent and adequately segregated. It shall be ensured that all left-overs of the previous packaging operations, including labels, cartons and caps are cleared before the closing hour.

Before packaging operations are begun, steps shall be taken to ensure that the work area, packaging lines, printing machines, and other equipment are clean and free from any products, materials and spillages. The line clearance shall be performed according to an appropriate checklist and recorded.

The correct details of any printing (for example of batch numbers or expiry dates) done separately or in the course of the packaging shall be re-checked at regular intervals. All printing and over-printing shall be authorised in writing.

The manufacturing environment shall be maintained at the required levels of temperature, humidity and cleanliness.

Authorised persons shall ensure change-over into specific uniforms before undertaking any manufacturing operations including packaging.

There shall be segregated secured areas for recalled or rejected material and for such material which are to be re-processed or recovered

All the materials & containers used in manufacturing process shall be conspicuously labeled with

- Name of product
- Batch number and batch size
- Stages of manufacture

9. Sanitation in manufacturing premises

The manufacturing premises shall be cleaned and maintained in an orderly manner, so that it is free from accumulated waste, dust, debris and other similar material. A validated cleaning procedure shall be maintained.
The manufacturing areas shall not be used for storage of materials, except for the material being processed. It shall not be used as a general thoroughfare.

A routine sanitation program shall be drawn up and observed, which shall be properly recorded and which shall indicate –

(a) specific areas to be cleaned and cleaning intervals

(b) cleaning procedure to be followed, including equipment and materials to be used for cleaning

(c) personnel assigned to and responsible for the cleaning operation. The adequacy of the working and in-process storage space shall permit the orderly and logical positioning of equipment and materials so as to minimise the risk of mix up between different pharmaceutical products or their components to avoid cross-contamination, and to minimise the risk of omission or wrong application of any of the manufacturing or control steps.

Production areas shall be well lit, particularly where visual on-line controls are carried out.

In short the above explanation can be summarized as follows:

- Manufacturing premises shall be Cleaned and maintained according to validated cleaning procedures.
- Manufacturing areas shall not be use as storage or thoroughfare
- A Routine sanitation program shall be drawn up and observed
- Area shall be well lightened production area particularly where visual on line controls carried out.

10. Raw materials

10.1. The licensee shall keep an inventory of all raw-materials to be used at any stage of manufacture of drugs and maintain records as per Schedule U.

All incoming materials shall be quarantined immediately after receipt or processing. All materials shall be stored under appropriate conditions and in an orderly fashion to permit batch segregation and stock rotation by a 'first in/first expiry' - 'first-out' principle. All incoming materials shall be checked to ensure that the consignment corresponds to the order placed.

All incoming materials shall be purchased from approved sources under valid purchase vouchers. Wherever possible, raw materials should be purchased directly from the producers.

Authorised staff appointed by the licensee in this behalf, which may include personnel from the quality control department, shall examine each consignment on receipt and shall check each container for integrity of package and seal. Damaged containers shall be identified, recorded and segregated.

If a single delivery of material is made up of different batches, each batch shall be considered as a separate batch for sampling, testing and release.

Raw materials in the storage area shall be appropriately labeled. Labels shall be clearly marked with the following information:

(a) Designated name of the product and the internal code reference, where applicable, and analytical reference number
(b) Manufacturer's name, address and batch number;
(c) The status of the contents (e.g. quarantine, under test, released, approved, rejected);
(d) The manufacturing date, expiry date and re-test date.

There shall be adequate separate areas for materials "under test", "approved", and "rejected" with arrangements and equipment to allow dry, clean and orderly placement of stored materials and products, wherever necessary, under controlled temperature and humidity.

Containers from which samples have been drawn shall be identified.

Only raw materials which have been released by the Quality Control Department and which are within their shelf-life shall be used. It shall be ensured that shelf life of formulation product shall not exceed with that of active raw materials used.

It shall be ensured that all the containers of raw materials are placed on the raised platforms/racks and not placed directly on the floor.

The licensee Keep an inventory of all raw materials to be used at any stage of production of drugs and maintain records as per Schedule U. All materials shall store under appropriate storage condition & follow 'first in/first expiry'– 'first out' rule. Raw material from each batch checked for quality & appropriately labels the storage area. There shall be adequate separate area for materials "under test", "approved", and "rejected" with arrangement and equipment.

It allow dry, clean and orderly placement of stored materials and products, wherever necessary, under controlled temp. and humidity. Only raw materials which have been released by the quality control department and which are within their shelf- life shall be used

It shall be ensured that shelf life of formulation product shall not exceed with that of active raw material used. It shall be ensured that all the containers of raw materials are placed on the raised platforms/racks and not placed directly on the floor.

11. Equipments

Equipment shall be located, designed, constructed, adapted and maintained to suit the operations to be carried out. The layout and design of the equipment shall aim to minimize the risk of errors and permit effective cleaning and maintenance in order to avoid cross- contamination, build –up of dust or dirt and in general any adverse effect on the quality of product.

Balance and other measuring equipment of an appropriate range, accuracy and precision shall be available in the raw material stores, production and in process control operation and these shall be calibrated and checked on a scheduled basis in accordance with SOP and record maintained.

To avoid accidental contamination, wherever possible, nontoxic/edible grade lubricant shall be used and the equipment shall be maintained in a way that lubricants don't Contaminate the products being produced.

Defective equipment shall be removed from production and quality control areas or appropriately labeled.

12. Documentation and records

It is the essential part of the Quality assurance system. as such , shall be Related to all aspect of GMP.

Its aim is to define the specification for all materials, method of manufacturing and control, to ensure that all personnel concerned with manufacture know the information necessary to decide whether or not to release a batch of a drug for sale and to provide an audit trail that shall permit investigation of the history of any suspected defective batch.

Documents shall be approved, signed and dated by appropriate and authorized persons.

Document designed, prepared, reviewed and controlled, wherever applicable, shall comply with these rules.

The records shall be made or completed at the time of each operation in such a way that all significant activities concerning the manufacturing of pharmaceutical product are traceable. Records and associate   SOP shall be retained for at least one year after the expiry date of the finished product.

13. Labels and other printed materials

Necessary for identification of the drugs and their use.

- Printed in bright colours and legible manner.
- All containers and equipment shall bear appropriate labels.
- Different color coded labels can be used.
- Printed packaging materials & leaflets shall be stored separately to avoid mix-up.
- Packaging, labeling and release shall be done after approval of QC department.
- Record of receipt and use of all material shall be maintained.

14. Quality assurance

To understand key issues in quality assurance/quality control.

To understand specific requirements on organization, procedures, processes and resources.

To develop actions to resolve current problems

Principles of Quality Assurance

Wide-ranging concept:

Covers all matters that individually or collectively

Influence the quality of a product. It is the totality of the arrangements made with the object of ensuring that the products are of the quality required for the intended use.

Quality Assurance incorporates GMP and also product design and development.

Requirements for QA Systems:

- Ensure products are developed correctly.
- Identify managerial responsibilities.
- Provide SOPs for production and control.
- Organize supply and use of correct starting materials.
- Define controls for all stages of manufacture and packaging.
- Ensure finished product correctly processed and checked before release
- Ensure products are released after review by authorized person
- Provide storage and distribution
- Organize self-inspection.

15. Self-inspection and Quality audit

It may be useful to constitute a self-inspection team supplemented with a quality audit procedure for assessment of all or part of a system with the specific purpose of improving it.

Ensures that a company's operations remain compliant with GMP.

Assists in ensuring continuous quality improvement.

Should cover all aspects of production and quality control which are designed to detect shortcomings in the implementation of GMP.

Must recommend corrective action if shortcomings are observed and set a timetable for corrective action to be completed.

Special occasions may demand additional self-inspections. For example,

- Recalls
- Repeated rejections
- GMP inspections announced by the National Drug Regulatory Authority.
- Written instructions for self-inspection include:
    (a)   Personnel
    (b)   Premises including personnel facilities
    (c)   Maintenance of buildings and equipment
    (d)   Storage of starting materials and finished
    (e)   Products
    (f)   Equipment
    (g)   Production and in-process controls
    (h)   Quality control
    (i)   Documentation
    (j)   Sanitation and hygiene

(k) Validation and revalidation programs

(l)   Calibration of instruments or measurement systems

(m) Recall procedures

(n) Complaints management

(o) Labels control

(p) Results of previous self-inspections and any corrective steps taken

Quality Audit

It may be useful to supplement self-inspection process with a quality audit. A quality audit consists of examination and assessment of all or part of a quality system with the specific purpose of improving it.

A quality audit is usually conducted by outside or independent specialist or a team designed by a management for this purpose. Such audits may also be conducted to suppliers and contractors. Basically three types: 1. Internal audit 2. External audit 3. Regulatory audit

16. Quality Control System

Quality control shall be concerned with sampling, specification, testing, documentation, and release procedures.

It is not confined to laboratory operations but shall be involved in all decisions concerning the quality of the product.

The department as a whole shall have other duties such as to establish, evaluate, validate and implement all Quality control procedure and methods.

All the batches released after certification of QC department.

Maintain reference/retained sample from each batch.

The area of the quality control laboratory may be divided into chemical, instrumentation ,microbiological and biological testing.

Adequate area having the required storage conditions shall be provided for keeping references samples. The quality control department shall evaluate, maintain and storage reference samples.

There shall be authorized and dated specifications for all materials, products, reagents.

The quality control department shall conduct stability studies of the products to ensure and assign their shelf life at the prescribed conditions of storage .All records of such studies shall be maintained.

The in charge of quality Assurance shall investigate all product complaints thereof shall be maintained

All instruments shall be calibrated and testing procedures validated before these are adopted for routine testing. Periodical calibration of instrument and validation of procedures shall be carried out.

Pharmacopoeias, reference standard, reference spectra, other references materials and technical books, as required, shall be available in the quality control laboratory of the licensee.

17. Specifications

17.1 For Raw materials and Packaging materials:- They shall include,-

(a)   the designated name and internal code reference;

(b)   reference, if any , to a pharmacopoeial monograph;

(c)   qualitative and quantitative requirements with acceptance limits;

(d)   name and address of manufacturer or supplier and original manufacturer of the material;

(e)   specimen of printed material;

(f)   directions for sampling and testing or reference to procedures;

(g)   storage conditions; and

(h)   Maximum period of storage before re-testing.

For Product Containers and Closures –

All containers and closures intended for use shall comply with the pharmacopoeial requirements. Suitable validated test methods, sample sizes, specifications, cleaning procedure and sterilization procedure, wherever indicated, shall be strictly followed to ensure that these are not reactive, additive, adsorptive, or leach to an extent that significantly affects the quality or purity of the drug. No second hand or used containers and closures shall be used.

Whenever bottles are being used, the written schedule of cleaning shall be laid down and followed. Where bottles are not dried after washing, they should be rinsed with de-ionised water or distilled water, as the case may be.

For in-process and bulk products. Specifications for in-process material, intermediate and bulk products shall be available. The specifications should be authenticated.

For Finished Products. Appropriate specifications for finished products shall include :

(a)   the designated name of the product and the code reference;

(b)   the formula or a reference to the formula and the pharmacopoeial reference;

(c)   directions for sampling and testing or a reference to procedures;

(d)   a description of the dosage form and package details;

(e)   the qualitative and quantitative requirements, with the acceptance limits for release;

(f)   the storage conditions and precautions, where applicable, and

(g)   the shelf-life.

For preparation of containers and closures. The requirements mentioned in the Schedule do not include requirements of machinery, equipments and premises required for preparation of containers and closures for different dosage forms and categories of drugs. The suitability and adequacy of the machinery, equipment and premises shall be examined taking into consideration the requirements of each licensee in this respect.

(a)   For raw material & packaging material.

(b)   For product containers & closures.

(c)   For in-process & bulk products.

(d)   For finished product

(e)   For preparation of containers & closures.

18.   Master formula records

There shall be Master Formula records relating to all manufacturing procedures for each product and batch size to be manufactured. These shall be prepared and endorsed by the competent technical staff i.e. head of production and quality control. The Master Formula shall include :-

A. The name of the product together with product reference code relating to its specifications

B. the patent or proprietary name of the product along with the generic name, a description of the dosage form, strength, composition of the product and batch size;

C. name, quantity, and reference number of all the starting materials to be used. Mention shall be made of any substance that may 'disappear' in the course of processing;

D. a statement of the expected final yield with the acceptable limits, and of relevant intermediate yields, where applicable;

E. a statement of the processing location and the principal equipment to be used;

F. The methods, or reference to the methods, to be used for preparing the critical equipment including cleaning, assembling, calibrating, sterilizing;

G. detailed stepwise processing instructions and the time taken for each step;

H. the instructions for in-process controls with their limits;

I. the requirements for storage conditions of the products, including the container, labelling and special storage conditions where applicable;

J. any special precautions to be observed;

K. packing details and specimen labels

Related to –

(a) All manufacturing procedures for each product.

(b) Batch size to be manufactured.

Includes:-

- Name of product with reference code
- Patent & proprietary name with generic name
- Description of dosage form.
- Name, quantity & reference no. Of all starting material.
- A statement of expected final yield & the principal equipment to be used.
- Detailed SOP with the time taken for each step.
- Requirements for storage conditions of the products, containers, labeling
- Packaging detail and specimen labels.

19. Packaging records

There shall be Authorized packaging instructions for each product, pack size & type that include;

- Name of product with other description.
- Volume of product in final container
- Complete list of all the packaging materials with.
- Quantities size & type.
- Description of packaging operations.
- Detail of in process control

20. Batch packaging record

A batch packaging record shall be kept for each batch or part batch processed. It shall be based on the relevant parts of packaging instructions, and the method of preparation of such records shall be designed to avoid transcription error.

Before any packaging operation begins, checks be made and recorded that the equipments and the work stations are clear of the previous products, documents or materials not required for the planned packaging operations, and that the equipment is clean and suitable for use.

21. Batch Processing Records

There shall be Batch processing Record for each product. It shall be based on the parts of the currently approved master formula. Before any processing begins, check shall be performed and recorded to ensure that the equipment and work station are clear of previous products, documents or materials not required for the planned process are removed and that equip0ment is clean an suitable for use.

During processing, the following information shall be recorded at the time each action is taken and the record shall be dated and signed by the person responsible for the processing operations:

- Name of the product
- No. of the batch being manufactured
- Date and time of commencement
- Initials of the operator of the different significant steps of production and where appropriate, of the person who checked each of these operations.
- Batch number.
- Equipments used.
- Records of the IPQC.
- Amount of then product obtained at different and critical stages of manufacture.
- Special problems

22. Standard operating procedures (SOP), and Records, Regarding.

22.1 Receipt of material Includes

- Written SOP for receipt of raw, primary & printed packaging materials.
- Written SOP for the internal labeling, quarantine & storage of various materials.
- SOPs for related instrument &equipment's.

22.2. Sampling Includes

- SOP for method of sampling.
- SOP for equipment's to be used.
- Precautions to avoid contamination.
- Instruction for qty. & pooling of sample.
- Specific precautions for sampling of sterile or hazardous materials

22.3. Batch numbering SOPs

Describing the detail of batch numbering set up for each batch of intermediate, bulk or finished product. Applied to a processing stage & to the respective packaging stage. Include date of allocation, product identity & batch size.

22.4 Testing

There shall be written procedures for testing materials and products at different stages of manufacture, describing the methods and equipment to be used, the tests performed shall be recorded.

23. Reference samples

Each lot of every active ingredient, in a quantity sufficient to carry out all the tests, except sterility and pyrogens/Bacterial Endotoxin test shall be retained for a period of 3 months after the date of expiry of the last batch produced from that active ingredient.

Samples of finished formulations shall be stored in the same or simulated containers in which the drug has been actually marketed.

24. Reprocessing and recording

Where processing is necessary, written procedures shall be established and approved by the Quality assurance Department that shall specify the condition and limitations of repeating chemical reactions. Such reprocessing shall be validated.

If the product batch has to be reprocessed the procedure shall be authorized and recorded. An investigation shall be carried out in to the causes necessitating reprocessed batch shall be subjected to stability evaluation

Recovery of product residue may be carried out, if permitted, in the master production and control records by incorporating it in subsequent batches of the product.

25. Distribution records

Prior to distribution or dispatch of given batch of a drug, it shall be ensured that the batch has been duly tested, approved and released by the quality control personnel. Pre-dispatch inspection shall be performed on each consignment on a random basis to ensure that only the correct goods are dispatched.

Records for distribution shall be maintained in a such manner that finished batch of a drug can be traced to the retail level to facilitate prompt and complete recall of the batch, if and when necessary.

26. Validation and Process Validation

Essential part of GMP and shall be conducted as per the pre–defined protocols.

A written report summarizing recorded result and conclusions shall be prepared, documented and maintained.

Shall be undergo periodic validation to ensure that they remain capable of achieving the intended results.

Critical process shall be validated, prospectively or retrospectively.

When any new master formula or method of preparation is adopted, steps shall be taken to demonstrate its suitability for routine processing.

Significant changes to the manufacturing Processes, including any change in equipment or materials that may affect product quality and/or the reproducibility of the process, shall be validated.

27. Product Recalls

A prompt and effective recall system of defective products shall be devised for timely information of all concerned stockists, wholesalers, suppliers, up to the retail level within the shortest period.

The licensee may make use of both print and electronic media in this regard

The distribution records shall be readily made available to the persons designated for recalls

The effectiveness of the arrangements for recalls shall be evaluated from time to time

The recalled products shall be stored separately in a secured segregated area pending final decision on them.

28. Complaints and Adverse Reactions

All complaints thereof concerning product quality shall be carefully reviewed and recorded according to written procedures. Each complaint shall be investigated /evaluated by the designated personnel of the company and records of investigation and remedial action taken thereof shall be maintained.

Reports of serious adverse drug reactions resulting from the use of a drug along with comments and documents shall be forthwith reported to the concerned Licensing Authority.

There shall be written procedures describing the action to be taken, recall to be made of the defective product.

29. Site Master File

The licensee shall prepare a succinct document in the form, of Site Master File Containing specific and factual GMP about the production and /or control of pharmaceutical manufacturing preparations carried out at the licensed premises.

A. General information
(a) Brief information of the firm
(b) Pharmaceutical manufacturing activities as permitted by the licensing authority
(c) Other manufacturing activities, if any, carried out on the premises
(d) Type of products licensed for manufacture with flowcharts mentioning procedures and process flow

(e) Number of employees engaged in the production, quality control, storage and distribution

(f) Use of outside scientific, analytical or other technical assistance in relation to manufacture and analysis

(g) Short description of the Quality Management system of the firm

(h) Products details registered with foreign countries.

B. Personnel

(a) Organizational chart showing the arrangement for quality assurance including production and quality control;

(b) qualification, experience and responsibilities of key personnel;

(c) outline for arrangements for basic and in-service training and how the records are maintained;

(d) health requirements for personal engaged in production

(e) Personnel hygiene requirements, including clothing.

C. Premises

(a) simple plan or description of manufacturing areas drawn to scale;

(b) nature of construction and fixtures / fittings;

(c) brief description of ventilation systems. More details should be given for critical areas with potential risk of airborne contamination (schematic drawing of systems). Classification of the rooms used for the manufacture of sterile products should be mentioned;

(d) special areas for the handling of the highly toxic, hazardous and sensitizing materials;

(e) brief description of water systems (schematic drawings of systems), including sanitation;

(f) Description of planned preventive maintenance programs for premises and of the recording system.

D. Equipment

(a) brief description of major equipment used in production and quality control laboratories (a list of equipment required);

(b) description of planned preventive maintenance programs for equipment and of the recording system;

(c) qualification and calibration, including the recording systems and arrangements for computerised systems validation.

E. Sanitation

(a) Availability of written specifications and procedures for cleaning manufacturing areas and equipment.

F. Documentation

(a)   Arrangements for the preparation, revision and distribution of document

(b)   necessary documentation for the manufacture;

(c)   any other documentation related to product quality that is not mentioned elsewhere (e.g. microbiological controls about air and water.

G. Production

(a)   brief description of production operations using, wherever possible, flow sheets and charts specifying important parameters;

(b)   arrangements for the handling of starting materials, packaging materials, bulk and finished products, including sampling, quarantine, release and storage;

(c)   arrangements for the handling of rejected materials and products;

(d)   brief description of general policy for process validation.

H. Quality control

(a)   Description of the quality control system and of the activities of the quality control department. Procedures for the release of the finished products.

(b)   Loan license manufacture and licensee

(c)   Description of the way in which compliance of Good Manufacturing Practices by the loan licensee shall be assessed.

(d)   Distribution, complaints and product recall

(e)   arrangements and recording system for distribution;

(f)   Arrangements for the handling of complaints and product recalls.

I. Self-Inspection

(a)   Short description of the self-inspection system indicating whether an outside, independent and experienced external expert was involved in evaluating the manufacturer's compliance with Good Manufacturing Practices in all aspects of production.

J. Export of drugs

(a)   products exported to different countries;

(b)   Complaints and product recall, if any.

FDA always ensures that the quality of drug products is not compromised by carefully monitoring drug manufacturers' compliance with its Current Good Manufacturing Practice (CGMP) regulations.

The CGMP regulations for drugs contain minimum requirements for the methods, facilities, and controls used in manufacturing, processing, and packing of a drug product. The regulations make sure that a product is safe for use, and that it has the ingredients and strength it claims to have.

The approval process for new and generic drug marketing applications includes a review of the manufacturer's compliance with the CGMPs. FDA assessors and investigators determine whether the firm has the necessary facilities, equipment, and ability to manufacture the drug it intends to market.

Change Control Format:

Introduction of New product and new Raw material

Product Name (If Any)	XYZ ... dosage Form
Market	Country Name :
Proposed Activity:	
Present Activity:	
Reason for Change	
Risk Analysis (attach approved Risk Analysis)	
Action of Risk analysis:	
Attachment (If Any)	Annexure I Annexure II

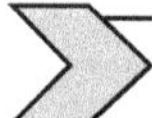

Important Questions

1. What is a GMP and CGMP? Why it is important for a Pharmaceutical company to comply with CGMP norms?

2. What are the important principles on which GMP rely?

3. What are the different parts of GMP?

4. Is a company required to notify the Inspectorate of a change in key personnel, such as the person in charge of Quality Control (QC) or manufacturing department?

5. Why separate areas are required for manufacturing facilities for contamination causing and potent products such as; β-lactam, sex hormones and cyto-toxic substance?

6. Packaging and Labelling form an important part of commercial product. Explain?

7. What is the importance of Ancillary areas? Explain.

8. Why quality control area and production area can't be merged together when they both form a part of any manufacturing unit? Explain.

9. Define Site master file. What are the content of site master file with advantages?

10. What is the difference between MFR and BMR?

11. What is the difference between MPR and BPR?

CHAPTER 3

Pharmaceutical Quality System - An Overview to ICH Q10 Guidelines

ICH Q10, PQS, is a guidance document first released for industry comment in June 2004, by the International Conference on Harmonisation of Technical Requirements for Registration of Pharmaceuticals for Human Use (ICH).

ICH Q10 is not intended to create new expectations beyond current regulatory requirements (such as PIC/S Guide to Good Manufacturing Practice for Medicinal Products) rather it helps to provide clarification, and is intended to be used alongside regulatory codes.

Objectives

ICH Q10 facilitates innovation and continual improvement throughout the product life cycle with three key objectives:

Achieve product realization that allows the delivery of quality products

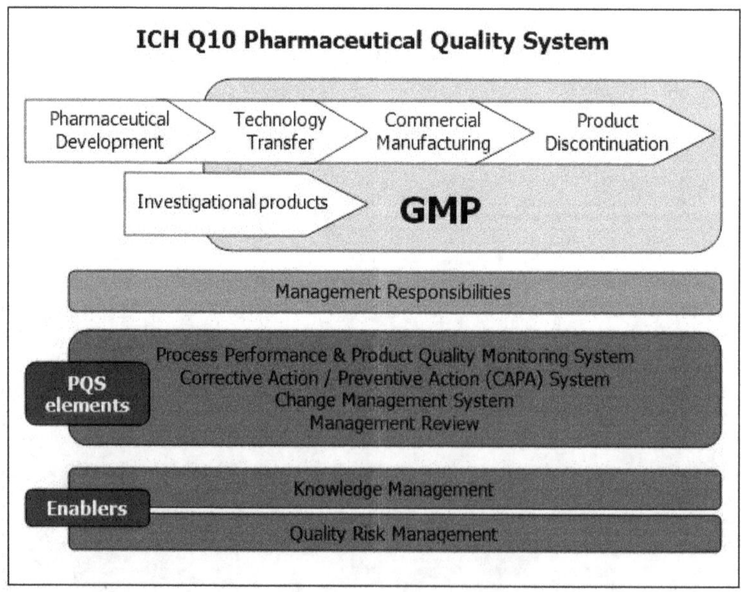

Flow chart showing pharmaceutical quality system

ICH Q10 includes practical guidance on the application of quality processes such as corrective and preventative actions (CAPA) and change management throughout your product lifecycle, helping to clarify the level of control required during development, scale-up, manufacturing through to discontinuation.

The elements of ICH Q10 should be applied in a manner that is appropriate and proportionate to each of the product lifecycle stages, recognizing the differences among, and the different goals of each stage.

The product lifecycle includes the following technical activities for new and existing products.

Pharmaceutical Development:

1. Drug substance development:

   Drug substance development and production is the foundation on which pharmaceutical product development is built. The ability to make consistent drug substance batches is key to turning a compound that shows promise in the laboratory into an effective and safe product.

2. **Formulation development (including container/closure system):**

   Drug formulation —also known as pharmaceutical formulation— is the process through which a variety of substances are combined with the drug's active pharmaceutical ingredient (API) to finally produce a drug product that can be successfully given to patients.

3. **Manufacture of investigational products:**

   Manufacturing drug products for clinical studies present many unique challenges that contrast to the manufacturing of commercial drug products. This article will explore the uniqueness of manufacturing IMPs (investigational medicinal products). Additionally, careful consideration will be paid to the planning phase and the challenges associated with manufacturing and packaging.

4. **Delivery system development (where relevant):**

   The systems development life cycle (SDLC) is a conceptual model used in project management that describes the stages involved in an information system development project, from an initial feasibility study through maintenance of the completed application. SDLC can apply to technical and non-technical systems.

5. **Manufacturing process development and scale-up:**

   A pilot plant can also be defined as the pre-commercial production system which includes new production technology and produces small volumes of new technology-based products scale-up is the process of increasing the batch size or a procedure for applying the same process to different output volumes.

6. Analytical method development.:

Pharmaceutical analysis plays a very prominent role in quality assurance as well as quality control of bulk drugs and pharmaceutical formulations. Rapid increase in pharmaceutical industries and production of drug in various parts of the world has brought a rise in demand for new analytical techniques in the pharmaceutical industries. As a consequence, analytical method development has become the basic activity of analysis. Recent development in analytical methods has been resulted from the advancement of analytical instruments.

Technology Transfer:

- New product transfers during Development through Manufacturing
- Transfers within or between manufacturing and testing sites for marketed products

Commercial Manufacturing:

- Acquisition and control of materials
- Provision of facilities, utilities, and equipment
- Production (including packaging and labelling)
- Quality control and assurance
- Release
- Storage
- Distribution (excluding wholesaler activities).

Product Discontinuation:

- Retention of documentation
- Sample retention
- Continued product assessment and reporting

Relationship of ICH Q10 to Regional GMP Requirements, ISO Standards and ICH Q7

Regional GMP requirements, the ICH Q7 Guideline, "Good Manufacturing Practice Guide for Active Pharmaceutical Ingredients", and ISO quality management system guidelines form the foundation for ICH Q10.

To meet the objectives described below, ICH Q10 augments GMPs by describing specific quality system elements and management responsibilities. ICH Q10 provides a harmonised model for a pharmaceutical quality system throughout the lifecycle of a product and is intended to be used together with regional GMP requirements.

The regional GMPs do not explicitly address all stages of the product lifecycle (e.g., Development). The quality system elements and management responsibilities described in this guideline are intended to encourage the use of science and risk based approaches at each lifecycle stage, thereby promoting continual improvement across the entire product lifecycle.

Relationship of ICH Q10 to Regulatory Approaches

Regulatory approaches for a specific product or manufacturing facility should be commensurate with the level of product and process understanding, the results of quality risk management, and the effectiveness of the pharmaceutical quality system. When implemented, the effectiveness of the pharmaceutical quality system can normally be evaluated during a regulatory inspection at the manufacturing site. Potential opportunities to enhance science and risk based regulatory approaches. Regulatory processes will be determined by region.

ICH Q10 Objectives:

- Achieve Product Realization
- Establish and Maintain a State of Control
- Facilitate Continual Improvement
- Enablers: Knowledge Management and Quality Risk Management
- Knowledge Management
- Quality Risk Management

Design and Content Considerations.

(a) The design, organization and documentation of the pharmaceutical quality system should be well structured and clear to facilitate common understanding and consistent application.

(b) The elements of ICH Q10 should be applied in a manner that is appropriate and proportionate to each of the product lifecycle stages, recognizing the different goals and knowledge available for each stage.

(c) The size and complexity of the company's activities should be taken into consideration when developing a new pharmaceutical quality system or modifying an existing one. The design of the pharmaceutical quality system should incorporate appropriate risk management principles. While some aspects of the pharmaceutical quality system can be company-wide and others site-specific, the effectiveness of the pharmaceutical quality system is normally demonstrated at the site level.

(d) The pharmaceutical quality system should include appropriate processes, resources and responsibilities to provide assurance of the quality of outsourced activities and purchased material.

(e) Management responsibilities, should be identified within the pharmaceutical quality system.

(f)   The pharmaceutical quality system should include the following elements,: process performance and product quality monitoring, corrective and preventive action, change management and management review.

(g)   Performance indicators, should be identified and used to monitor the effectiveness of processes within the pharmaceutical quality system.

Quality Manual

Quality Manual or equivalent documentation approach should be established and should contain the description of the pharmaceutical quality system. The description should include:

(a)   The quality policy

(b)   The scope of the pharmaceutical quality system

(c)   Identification of the pharmaceutical quality system processes, as well as their sequences, linkages and interdependencies. Process maps and flow charts can be useful tools to facilitate depicting pharmaceutical quality system processes in a visual manner

(d)   Management responsibilities within the pharmaceutical quality system.

Management Responsibility

Leadership is essential to establish and maintain a company-wide commitment to quality and for the performance of the pharmaceutical quality system.

Management Commitment

(a)   Senior management has the ultimate responsibility to ensure an effective pharmaceutical quality system is in place to achieve the quality objectives, and that roles, responsibilities, and authorities are defined, communicated and implemented throughout the company.

(b)   Management should:

(i)   Participate in the design, implementation, monitoring and maintenance of an effective pharmaceutical quality system

(ii)   Demonstrate strong and visible support for the quality of Pharmaceutical system and ensure its implementation throughout their organization;

(iii)   Ensure a timely and effective communication and escalation process exists to raise quality issues to the appropriate levels of management;

(iv)   Define individual and collective roles, responsibilities, authorities and inter-relationships of all organisational units related to the pharmaceutical quality system. Ensure these interactions are communicated and understood at all levels of the organisation. An independent quality unit/structure with authority to fulfil certain pharmaceutical quality system responsibilities is required by regional regulations.

(v) Conduct management reviews of process performance and product quality and of the pharmaceutical quality system

(vi) Advocate continual improvement

(vii) Commit appropriate resources.

Quality Policy

(a) Senior management should establish a quality policy that describes the overall intentions and direction of the company related to quality.

(b) The quality policy should include an expectation to comply with applicable regulatory requirements and should facilitate continual improvement of the pharmaceutical quality system.

(c) The quality policy should be communicated to and understood by personnel at all levels in the company.

(d) The quality policy should be reviewed periodically for continuing effectiveness.

Quality Planning

(a) Senior management should ensure the quality objectives needed to implement the quality policy are defined and communicated.

(b) Quality objectives should be supported by all relevant levels of the company.

(c) Quality objectives should align with the company's strategies and be consistent with the quality policy.

(d) Management should provide the appropriate resources and training to achieve the quality objectives.

(e) Performance indicators that measure progress against quality objectives should be established, monitored, communicated regularly and acted upon.

Resource Management

(a) Management should determine and provide adequate and appropriate resources (human, financial, materials, facilities and equipment) to implement and maintain the pharmaceutical quality system and continually improve its effectiveness.

(b) Management should ensure that resources are appropriately applied to a specific product, process or site.

Internal Communication

(a) Management should ensure appropriate communication processes are established and implemented within the organisation.

(b) Communications processes should ensure the flow of appropriate information between all levels of the company.

(c) Communication processes should ensure the appropriate and timely escalation of certain product quality and pharmaceutical quality system issues.

Management Review

(a) Senior management should be responsible for pharmaceutical quality system governance through management review to ensure its continuing suitability and effectiveness.

(b) Management should assess the conclusions of periodic reviews of process performance and product quality and of the pharmaceutical quality system.

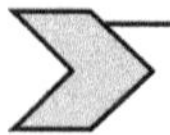

Continual Improvement of Process Performance and Product Quality

This section describes the lifecycle stage goals and the four specific pharmaceutical quality system elements that augment regional requirements to achieve the ICH Q10 objectives, It does not restate all regional GMP requirements.

Lifecycle Stage Goals

The goals of each product lifecycle stage are described below

Pharmaceutical Development

The goal of pharmaceutical development activities is to design a product and its manufacturing process to consistently deliver the intended performance and meet the needs of patients and healthcare professionals, and regulatory authorities and internal customers' requirements. Approaches to pharmaceutical development are described in ICH Q8. The results of exploratory and clinical development studies, while outside the scope of this guidance, are inputs to pharmaceutical development.

Technology Transfer

The goal of technology transfer activities is to transfer product and process knowledge between development and manufacturing, and within or between manufacturing sites to achieve product realisation. This knowledge forms the basis for the manufacturing process, control strategy, process validation approach and ongoing continual improvement

Commercial Manufacturing

The goals of manufacturing activities include achieving product realisation, establishing and maintaining a state of control and facilitating continual improvement. The pharmaceutical quality system should assure that the desired product quality is routinely met, suitable process performance is achieved, the set of controls are appropriate, improvement opportunities are identified and evaluated, and the body of knowledge is continually expanded.

Product Discontinuation

The goal of product discontinuation activities is to manage the terminal stage of the product lifecycle effectively. For product discontinuation, a pre-defined approach should be used to manage activities such as retention of documentation and samples and continued product assessment (e.g., complaint handling and stability) and reporting in accordance with regulatory requirements.

Pharmaceutical Quality System Elements

The elements described below might be, required in part under regional GMP regulations. However, the Q10 model's intent is to enhance these elements in order to promote the lifecycle approach to product quality. These four elements are:

Process performance and product quality monitoring system;

Corrective action and preventive action (CAPA) system;

Change management system;

Management review of process performance and product quality.

These elements should be applied in a manner that is appropriate and proportionate to each of the product lifecycle stages, recognizing the differences among, and the different goals of, each stage. Throughout the product lifecycle, companies are encouraged to evaluate opportunities for innovative approaches to improve product quality.

Monitoring of Internal and External Factors Impacting the Pharmaceutical Quality System Factors monitored by management can include:

(a) Emerging regulations, guidance and quality issues that can impact the Pharmaceutical Quality System;

(b) Innovations that might enhance the pharmaceutical quality system;

(c) Changes in business environment and objectives;

(d) Changes in product ownership

Outcomes of Management Review and Monitoring

The outcome of management review of the pharmaceutical quality system and monitoring of internal and external factors can include:

(a) Improvements to the pharmaceutical quality system and related processes;

(b) Allocation or reallocation of resources and/or personnel training;

(c) Revisions to quality policy and quality objectives

(d) Documentation and timely and effective communication of the results of the management review and actions, including escalation of appropriate issues to senior management.

The International Conference on Harmonization ICH Q10 guideline, *Pharmaceutical Quality System*, and its two companion guidelines Q8 *Pharmaceutical Development* and Q9 *Quality Risk Management*, have been readily accepted, if not fully implemented by the pharmaceutical industry over the past few years.

Generic industry aims to produce safe, efficient, built-in quality medicines that will satisfy patients' requirements and will be competitive on the market. The review of the guidelines indicates differences in the life cycle of a generic medicine, leading to a final conclusion in terms of generic industry.

PAT provides statistical analysis and real time quality monitoring, as the basis for proactive quality management. Using QbD/PAT, quality is proved and improved throughout the entire life cycle.

Better understanding of the product and processes within a defined design space leads to easier proof of built-in quality throughout the life cycle of the medicine, faster and easier regulatory evaluation, faster time to market, as well as post marketing savings regarding costs and time.

Implementation of QbD/PAT as a systematic approach together with risk assessment as part of quality management system is a useful challenge to the generic industry and gives an opportunity for technological, temporal, financial and quality improvement.

It was concluded that having in mind its' own manufacturing capabilities the applicant should optimize the implementation of QbD in accordance with current good manufacturing practice guidelines. Implementation of QbD/PAT is an innovative challenge for the generic industry.

Managing pharmaceutical quality system allows the top management to make right decisions at the right time.

The goal is to recognize the benefits, challenges and opportunities deriving from implementation of the guidelines, including Quality by design (QbD) and Process analytical technology (PAT), from a critical viewpoint of the generic pharmaceutical industry related to the regulation and authorities evaluation of the application, concerning medicine quality.

The empirical approach is based on predefined specification that available data should comply with. Determination of one variable at a time may end up with Out of Specification results, leading to quarantine or withdrawal of the product.

Controls of materials and processes are repeated after each cycle, production process is fixed, without possibility of unauthorized changes, and its validation is based on minimum three pilot batches manufactured at industrial facilities.

The control strategy is out of site testing and inspection, focused on repeatability and optimization of processes, controlled in terms of specification approved with the Marketing Authorization (MA). Retrospective quality assurance and corrective measures, based on in-process and finished product analysis are used, where opportunities for statistical and basic problem cause analysis are limited (ICH Q8, 2008).

On the other hand ICH Q10 gives guidance for implementation and management of modern quality system. While it doesn't talk for a specific product but for the system as a whole, however, the focus is on specific measurements of product and processes quality that demonstrate continuous improvement of the realized product, that should satisfy consumers' quality requirements.

ICH Q10 provides management of changes within the design space. Any successfully designed pharmaceutical quality system contains elements of risk management (ICH Q9, 2005). From this it can be concluded that to enjoy the benefits of implementing ICH Q8 and ICH Q9 implementation of ICH Q10 cannot be avoided.

For successful implementation of QbD and PAT, the industry should follow the directions given in the guidelines ICH Q8, Q9, Q10.

Because of the rigorous requirements set for the manufacturing processes, the pharmaceutical industry is far behind other industries in terms of improving the techniques and processes for on line control.On the other hand, regulators require following of new technology achievements, and the PAT represents a chance for the pharmaceutical industry to bring innovation in the development and control of manufacturing process.

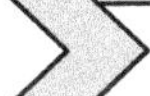 **Important Questions**

1. Why do we need a modern pharmaceutical quality system?

2. What is the purpose of ICH Q 10? Explain.

3. Briefly explain the scope of ICH Q10?

4. What is the relationship between ICH Q10 and regional GMP'S.?

5. Briefly explain the design and content of ICH Q10?

6. What are the key elements of ICH Q10?

7. A modern pharmaceutical quality system needs to be holistic and cover the product lifecycle. Explain?

8. How continual improvement in the pharmaceutical quality management can be obtained through ICH Q10?

9. Why do we need a modern pharmaceutical quality system?

CHAPTER 4

Analysis of Corrective and Preventive Action

Troubleshooting problems and attempting to identify and prevent potential problems is a typical activity for most businesses. The reason is obvious. Problems have a financial impact on the company. The ability to correct existing problems or implementing controls to prevent potential problems is essential for continued customer satisfaction and efficient business practice.

However, the missing link in this process is often adequate documentation of the actions taken. Properly documented actions provide important historical data for a continuous quality improvement plan and are essential for any product that must meet regulatory requirements demanded by FDA and ISO and other quality systems.

This is the reason for the implementation of a formal Corrective Action / Preventive Action (CAPA) program. CAPA is a major area of concern for both FDA, ISO 9000, as well as the Automotive and Aerospace industries. They have recognized that how a quality system is maintained and monitored is critical to its effectiveness.

Their risk-based CAPA requirements demand a well documented system that determines the root cause of nonconformance's, system failures, or process problems, corrects the problems, and prevents them from recurring.

The documentation must identify why something went (or may go) wrong and what has been done to make sure it does not happen again CAPA is a fundamental management tool that should be used in every quality system. This program provides a simple step by step process for completing and documenting corrective or preventive actions.

The result will be a complete, well documented investigation and solution that will satisfy regulatory requirements and form the basis for an effective continuous improvement plan for any company.

What is CAPA

CAPA is Corrective and Preventive actions, however it is much more than just "Corrective actions" and "Preventive actions".

Corrective Action

is the action to eliminate the cause of a detected nonconformity or other undesirable situation and Preventive Action is the action to eliminate the cause of a potential nonconformity or other undesirable potential situation. The process includes:

- Reviewing and defining the problem or nonconformity
- Finding the cause of the problem
- Developing an action plan to correct the problem and prevent a recurrence
- Implementing the plan
- Evaluating the effectiveness of the correction.

Preventive Actions

A preventive action is a process for detecting potential problems or nonconformance's and eliminating them. The process includes:

- Identify the potential problem or nonconformance
- Find the cause of the potential problem
- Develop a plan to prevent the occurrence.
- Implement the plan
- Review the actions taken and the effectiveness in preventing the problem.

Differences between Corrective and Preventive Actions

The process used for corrective actions and preventive actions is very similar and the steps outlined in this document can be used for either.

However, it is important to understand the differences and also be aware of the implications involved in performing and documenting each.

A corrective action is a reaction to a problem that has already occurred. It assumes that a nonconformance or problem exists and has been reported by either internal or external sources. The actions initiated are intended to:

(a) Fix the problem

(b) Modify the quality system so that the process that caused it is monitored to prevent a reoccurrence.

The documentation for a corrective action provides evidence that the problem was recognized, corrected, and proper controls installed to make sure that it does not happen again. For example, in a manufacturing setting, a large batch of subassemblies produced four weeks ago was found to be out of specification when received for final product assembly.

In this situation a problem exists and has been identified. A corrective action must be implemented to avoid production delays and a possible financial impact on the company.

A preventive action is initiated to stop a potential problem from occurring. It assumes that adequate monitoring and controls are in place in the quality system to assure that potential problems are identified and eliminated before they happen.

If something in the quality system indicates that a possible problem is or may develop, a preventive action must be implemented to avert and then eliminate the potential situation.

The documentation for a preventive action provides evidence that an effective quality system has been implemented that is able to anticipate, identify and eliminate potential problems.

CAPA is vital to an organization's regulatory compliance initiatives. An effective CAPA program will decrease process variation and improve product quality. The source of CAPA is critical to understand, depends on the criticality the priority can be decided.

Management support and management review are necessary for an effective CAPA process. CAPA methodology must result in product and process improvements and enhanced product and process understanding.

CAPA Procedures

Implementing an effective corrective or preventive action capable of satisfying quality assurance and regulatory documentation requirements is accomplished in seven basic steps:

1. The Identification of the problem, nonconformity, or incident or the potential problem,
2. Non conformity, or incident.
3. An Evaluation of the magnitude of the problem and potential impact on the company.
4. The development of an Investigation procedure with assignments of responsibility.
5. Performing a thorough Analysis of the problem with appropriate documentation
6. Creating an Action Plan listing all the tasks that must be completed to correct and/or prevent the problem.
7. The Implementation the plan.
8. A thorough Follow up with verification of the completion of all tasks, and an assessment of the appropriateness and effectiveness of the actions taken

Challenges of CAPA Management System

Improper investigation of the cause resulting from different quality systems

Recurring issues because of unstructured fixing of the problems.

Focusing on remedial action to run the business.

Insufficient management review on Quality Management System.

Lack of resources and competency.

More focus on manufacturing activities for more output.

More reactive approach than proactive.

Attributes of CAPA Management System

The main aspects of CAPA management system are assigning the CAPA, monitoring the CAPA progress and the effectiveness check of CAPA.

Assigning the CAPA

It is the very basic step to mitigate the non compliance issues. One has to identify correct root cause of issue, once the root cause is identified it become easier to assign corrective action and preventive action which will take care of identified issue to avoid recurrence and potential issue to avoid occurrence respectively.

Many organizations are failed at this step which invites the recurrence of the same issue again and again. The reason behind the recurrence is improper investigation of non compliance issues. There are various methods or tools that provide correct investigation of issue for example Fish bone analysis, Failure mode effective analysis and 5 Why's etc. Correct follow up of investigation tool will give you correct root cause that contribute assigning the precise and accurate CAPA.

Monitoring the CAPA Progress

Now days in market various software, tools and techniques are available to monitor the progress of CAPA. The ultimate significance of these software, tools and techniques is to monitor the completion of the defined actions and respect the timelines of those actions. The advanced software like SAP, Trackwise are readily available solution which is easily configured to fit business processes without the need for customization. However some organizations are still using the ERP modules or Spreadsheet to monitor the progress of CAPA. Mitigation of actions and catching the timelines are crucial rather than having the best software or ERP module.

Effectiveness check of CAPA

It is not always necessary that once the CAPA has been given there will not be recurrence of the issue. The same issue may trigger because of another reason. Effectiveness check of CAPA is essential so as to verify with implemented CAPA, there is compliance, improved control, and reduced risk of recurrence and lower costs through the consolidation of redundant systems. Effectiveness check can be done by revisiting the actions that has been implemented so as to comply the non -conformities.

Centralized CAPA Management and Sources of CAPA

A mature quality management system detects the problems before they occur and then prevent the problems. CAPA is of paramount importance to the FDA. According to FDA documents CAPA accounts for 30-50% of FDA-483 forms issued for non compliance.

All the elements of quality management system that are different quality systems to oversight business processes must have their own management systems. Failure of these systems indicates the business processes are not followed. The business processes falls under the Tier 1 which are for different operational activities.

For e.g. day in and day out activities of production floor and QC laboratories. The quality systems falls under the Tier 2 that governs the business process. Failure to business processes will definitely fail the quality systems.

The CAPA management system governs the Tier 2 to have better control to be in compliance with regulatory and cGMP. Internal audit management system is verification of compliance by self, so it is very useful for the organization to identify the gaps and mitigate before it is noticed by external regulatory agency.

This system is prime source of CAPA and provides the oversight on business processes so that organization can meet cGMP and regulatory requirement. Customer complaint management is crucial to any Pharmaceutical organization as it involves health of customer and reputation and cost of the organization.

Therefore the CAPA resulting from the customer complaint has to mitigate on priority. Deviations management is one more source of the CAPA. Deviation system manages the unplanned events which may have occurred due to malfunctioning of the operation, machines etc. Basically deviations are nothing but the diversion of defined standard procedure. CAPA resulting from deviations are more concerned of FDA inspectors as the deviations are not the usual thing. Change control is another system where planned event are captured, the CAPA resulting from the change control system is to be focused consciously because the change executed has to be verified for its successful implementation.

Risk Management is one of the very essential quality systems to run the business successfully. This system provides the futuristic events that may trouble the organization by achieving the strategic goals. So the CAPA resulting from risk management is beneficial to business to avoid the issues proactively.

Recall system is also important source of critical CAPA where organization has direct connection with regulatory agencies. What actions need to be taken to avoid the recall because of same cause. Regulatory inspection is one of the major sources of CAPA and be follow closely to avoid further non compliances. In addition to these sources of CAPA one of the important aspects is the annual product review. In annual product review whatever actions arising need to consider as part of continues improvement of the quality management system.

CAPA is at the center for controlling the effectiveness of quality management system to drive organizational efficiencies and modernization with respect to compliance status of organization.

Benefits of the Centralized CAPA Management

- Fulfills the promise of continuous improvement
- Leads to better customer satisfaction and less risk to the public.
- Better use of resources through a structured QA system.
- Facilitate better and more informed decisions by organizations.
- Makes good business and financial sense
- Increasing organization's compliance quotient.
- A reduction in quality and severity of issues
- More preventive actions over time
- Better designed products/processes.
- Improved customer satisfaction.

Better business results In addition to above benefits, the organization is always in a status of compliance and can be said as all time readiness for inspection with proper implementation of CAPA. Implementing a centralize CAPA management system as part of an overall quality management has ultimately reduced costs and enhance the growth of organization.

CAPA system is center of the quality management system where all the actions are narrowed down. Effective collection of these actions resulting from the non compliances of quality system will help organization to avoid non compliances and ultimately reduced the FDA citation.

CAPA management system regulates the non compliance by finding out root cause of the issue, defining the actions, following the actions till mitigation, effectiveness of action for continuous improvement. Effectiveness of the actions must undergo to management review which would complete the closed loop of CAPA management system.

The centralized CAPA management system must avoid the non-compliances when used with correct approach. This will save the time, money and resources of the organizations.

CAPA Procedures

Implementing an effective corrective or preventive action capable of satisfying quality assurance and regulatory documentation requirements is accomplished in seven basic steps:

- The identification of the problem, nonconformity, or incident or the potential problem, nonconformity, or incident.

- An evaluation of the magnitude of the problem and potential impact on the company.

- The development of an investigation procedure with assignments of responsibility.

- Performing a thorough analysis of the problem with appropriate documentation.

- Creating an action plan listing all the tasks that must be completed to correct and/or prevent the problem.

- The implementation the plan.

A thorough Follow up with verification of the completion of all tasks, and an assessment of the appropriateness and effectiveness of the actions taken

Note: There are an extensive number of variables in any process whether it is manufacturing, software development, or technical services that have the ability to generate occasional quality problems, nonconformities or adverse incidents.

These may be actual events that have occurred or circumstances that have the potential to cause a future nonconformance. For the purpose of this program these events or potential events will be referred to as "problems." Identification

The initial step in the process is to clearly define the problem. It is important to accurately and completely describe the situation as it exists now. This should include the source of the information, a detailed explanation of the problem, the available evidence that a problem exists.

Documenting the source of the information can be very useful when conducting an investigation into the problem and implementing the action plan that is created. It will also provide data for evaluating the effectiveness of the quality system and facilitate communicating the completion of the action to the appropriate individuals or departments.

This information may come from many possible sources. For example, situations that require corrective actions may come from external sources such as customer concerns or service requests. Internal quality audits, staff observations, quality assurance inspections, trending data, and management review are all examples of possible internal sources of information.

Examples of sources that lead to preventive actions may include: Service Request, Internal Quality Audit, Customer Complaint / Concern, Quality Assurance Inspection, Staff Observation, Trending Data Risk Assessment, Process Performance Monitoring, Management Review, Failure Mode Analysis and other sources are possible and will depend on the circumstances.

Explanation of the Problem

A complete description of the problem is written. The description should be concise but must contain sufficient information to assure that the problem can be easily understood from reading the explanation.

Evidence List the specific information available that demonstrates that the problem does exist. For example, the evidence for a product defect may be a high percentage of service requests or product returns. The evidence for a potential equipment problem may be steadily increasing downtime.

Corrective/Preventive Action Request form

A sample form is provided "Corrective/Preventive Action Request that can be used to initiate a CAPA action and collect the initial information.

Evaluation

The situation that has been described and documented in the "Identification" section should now be evaluated to determine first, the need for action and then the level of action required. The potential impact of the problem and the actual risks to the company and/or customers must be determined.

Essentially, the reasons that this problem is a concern must be documented.

Potential Impact

Part of the evaluation is a specific explanation of specifically why the problem is a concern. This may include the possible impact that the problem may have in terms of costs, function, product quality, safety, reliability, and customer satisfaction.

Assessment of Risk

Using the result of the impact evaluation, the seriousness of the problem is assessed. The level of risk that is associated with the problem may affect the actions that are taken. For example, a problem that presents a serious risk to the function or safety of a product may be assigned a high priority and require immediate remedial action.

On the other hand, an observation that a particular machine is experiencing an increasing level of downtime each month may have a lower priority.

Remedial Action

Based on the outcome of the impact and risk evaluations above, it may be determined that immediate remedial action is required to remedy the situation until a thorough investigation and a permanent solution is implemented.

If remedial actions are necessary, the actions and the resources required are listed. The steps that must be taken immediately to avoid any further adverse effects are explained. The actions that are taken are documented. This documentation will become part of the 'Action Implementation' and 'Follow Up' sections of the CAPA action.

In some instances it may be determined that the remedial action is all that is needed. In that case, a rationale is written for that decision, appropriate follow up is done, and the CAPA closed out.

Remedial Action form

This form should be used to explain the steps that must be taken to avoid any further adverse effects.

Investigation

In this step of the process a procedure is written for conducting an investigation into the problem. A written plan helps assure that the investigation is complete and nothing is missed. The procedure should include: an objective for the actions that will be taken, the procedure to be followed, the personnel that will be responsible, and any other anticipated resources needed.

Objective

The first step in the investigation is to state an objective for the action. In the "Identification" section the problem was defined and the current situation stated. The objective is a statement of the desired outcome of the corrective or preventive action.

State what the situation will be when the action is complete. This may be a statement in the form of: "the problem will be corrected, all effects of the problem identified and rectified, and controls will be in place to prevent the situation from happening again.

Investigation Procedure

A set of specific instructions are created that outline what must be done to determine the contributing and root cause of the problem. The investigation procedure will vary depending on the circumstances, but must incorporate a comprehensive review and analysis of all of the circumstances related to the problem. Consider equipment, materials, personnel, procedures, design, training, software, and external factors.

Responsibilities / Resources

An important part of the investigation procedure is to assign responsibility for conducting each aspect of the investigation. Any additional resources that may be required is also identified and documented. For example, specific testing equipment or external analysis may be required.

Investigation Procedure form

This is a written plan of action for the investigation into the problem. It should include the overall objective and the instructions for conducting the investigation. The person or persons responsible for the investigation and an expected completion date should also be entered.

Analysis

The investigation procedure that was created is now used to investigate the cause of the problem. The goal of this analysis is primarily to determine the root cause of the problem described, but any contributing causes are also identified. This process involves collecting relevant data, investigating all possible causes, and using the information available to determine the cause of the problem.

It is very important to distinguish between the observed symptoms of a problem and the fundamental root cause of the problem.

Note: There are many formal methods of performing root cause analysis. A discussion of specific methods is beyond the scope of this book.

Possible Causes / Data Collection

A list of all possible causes is created. This will form the basis for collecting relevant information, test data, etc. For example, consider the situation where a large batch of parts from a CNC Mill was discovered to be out of tolerance. There are many possible causes for this condition including: operator error, incorrect software, a dull or broken tool, an incorrect or obsolete print, a material problem, a design problem, etc.

By considering all possible causes, appropriate information and data can be collected that will be ultimately be used to determine the root cause of the problem.

Results and Data

The results of the data collection are documented and organized. This may include a combination of testing results and/or a review of records, processes, service information, design controls, operations, and any other data that may lead to a determination of the fundamental cause of the problem.

The resulting documentation should be complete and address all of the possible causes that were previously determined. This information is used to determine the root cause of the problem.

Root Cause Analysis

Determining the root cause often requires answering a series of 'why?' questions and digging deep into the situation until the fundamental reason for the problem is found. For example, in the out of tolerance parts situation described earlier, the investigation revealed that the operator had not been properly trained and had forgotten an essential step in the machining process.

The improperly trained operator is the immediate cause of the problem, but may not be the root cause. Why was the operator not trained properly? Are the existing training programs adequate and are they being implemented properly? Further investigation revealed that the operator was on vacation when the training was given and, therefore, did not receive the training when other operators did. The root cause of the problem was a lack of follow up in the training program.

No mechanism existed to cross check training records to assure that a missed training session was rescheduled. The root cause of the problem is documented. This will be essential for determining the appropriate corrective and/or preventive actions that must be taken.

Problem Analysis form

A sample "Problem Analysis" form is included. This form is optional but is intended to be used for recording information related to the analysis of the problem. The form can be used as a collection point for the information discovered during the analysis and any supporting data or documentation can be attached.

Action Plan

By using the results from the Analysis, the optimum method for correcting the situation (or preventing a future occurrence) is determined and an action plan developed. The plan should include, as appropriate: the items to be completed, document changes, any process, procedure, or system changes required, employee training, and any monitors or controls necessary to prevent the problem or a recurrence of the problem.

The action plan should also identify the person or persons responsible for completing each task.

Actions to be Complete

List all of the activities and tasks that must be accomplished to either correct the existing problem or eliminate a potential problem. For a CAPA program to be effective, it is very important to take a very global approach. Make sure to identify all actions that will be required to address everything related to the situation.

For example, in the training situation described earlier, the root cause was a flaw in the training program. One of the actions that must be taken is to review all previous training records to determine if this problem resulted in any other employee not receiving necessary training.

Document or Specification changes

List any documents that will be modified and describe in general terms what the modifications will be.

Process, Procedure, or System changes

If any changes to processes, procedures, or systems must be made they are described. Enough detail should be included so that it is clearly understood what must be done. The expected outcome of these changes should also be explained.

Employee Training

Employee training is an essential part of any change that is made and should be part of the action plan. To assure that the actions taken will be effective, any modifications made to documents, processes, etc. must be effectively communicated to all persons or departments that will be affected.

Action Plan form

This should provide a set of written procedures that detail all of the actions that must be done to resolve the problem and prevent it from recurring. This includes corrective and preventive activities, document changes, training, etc. The person or persons responsible and an expected completion date should also be entered on the form

Action Implementation

The corrective / preventive action plan that has been created is now implemented. All of the required tasks listed and described in the action plan are initiated, completed, and documented.

Implementation Summary

All of the activities that have been completed as required in the "Action Plan" should be listed and summarized. This section should contain a complete record of the actions that were taken to correct the problem and assure that it will not recur. This includes changes, preventive measures, process controls, training, etc. Documentation All documents or other specifications that have been modified are listed. Typically the documentation would be attached to a final printed report of this CAPA action. This will facilitate verification of the changes for the follow up.

Follow Up

One of the most fundamental steps in the CAPA process is an evaluation of the actions that were taken. Several key questions must be answered:

1. Have all of the objectives of this CAPA been met? (Did the actions correct or prevent the problem and are there assurances that the same situation will not happen again?)
2. Have all recommended changes been completed and verified.
3. Has appropriate communications and training been implemented to assure that all relevant employees understand the situation and the changes that have been made?
4. Is there any chance that the actions taken may have had any additional adverse effect on the product or service?

Verification Results

The implementation and completion of all changes, controls, training, etc. must be verified. The evidence that this has been done must be recorded. Appropriate information should have been entered to document that all actions have been completed successfully.

Results / Effectiveness of the Actions

Another important aspect of any CAPA action is to make sure that the actions taken were effective. A thorough evaluation must be done to make sure that the root cause of the problem has been solved, that any resulting secondary situations have been corrected, that proper controls have been established, and that adequate monitoring of the situation is in place. This evaluation must also include an investigation to determine if the actions taken could result in any other adverse effects. This investigation and the results should be documented.

Additional Comments

It is always a good idea to add any additional information or other appropriate comments concerning the problem, investigation, actions, or follow up that may be helpful in understanding anything that has been done for a CAPA action.

Documenting the complete process involved in a corrective or preventive action from identifying the problem to a successful completion is important for all companies, but absolutely essential for meeting current regulatory requirements.

Following the steps outlined in this document will provide a complete, well documented CAPA action that will meet regulatory requirements and can significantly improve the quality process in an organization. When the Follow up is complete, there should be a formal indication that it has been completed

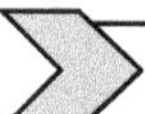 **Important Questions**

1. What should really trigger CAPA?

2. What is the difference between corrective and preventive actions?

3. Briefly explain the challenges associated with CAPA?

4. What are the attributes of CAPA management system?

5. How recall system is critical to CAPA?

6. Enlist the procedure required for carrying out effective CAPA?

7. Determine how root cause analysis is done through CAPA?

8. An important aspect of any CAPA action is to make sure that the actions taken were effective. Explain?

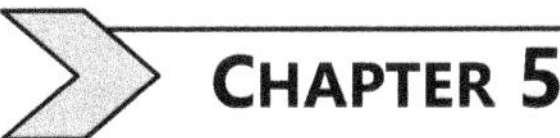

CHAPTER 5

Assuring Pharmaceutical Quality- A Brief Analysis of SOP's

A quality system is defined as the organizational structure, responsibilities, processes, procedures and resources for implementing quality management. Quality management includes those aspects of the overall management function that determine and implement the company quality policy and quality objectives. Both quality control and quality assurance are parts of quality management.

The 13th principle in the International Conference on Harmonization Good Clinical Practice (ICH GCP) guideline clearly states that systems and procedures that assure the quality of every aspect of the clinical trial should be implemented.

The sponsor is responsible for implementing and maintaining quality assurance and quality control systems with written SOPs to ensure that trials are conducted and data are generated, documented (recorded) and reported in compliance with the protocol, Good Clinical Practice (GCP) and the applicable regulatory requirements.

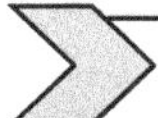

Standard Operating Procedures

Standardization is defined as an activity that gives rise to solutions for repetitive application to problems in various disciplines including science and it is aimed at achieving the optimum degree of order in a given context. Generally, the activity consists of the process of establishing (determining, formulating, and issuing) and implementing standards. Therefore, standards are the ultimate result of a standardization activity and within the context of quality systems consist of quality documents or documents related to the quality systems.

The quality documents consist of Company policies, quality management plan, SOPs, working instructions, conventions, guidelines, forms, templates, logs, tags and labels. They are established by consensus and approved by a nominated body and they provide for common and repeated use, rules, guidelines or characteristics for activities or their results with a view to promote transparency, consistency, reproducibility, interchangeability and to facilitate communication. The hierarchy and types of quality documents relevant to quality systems will depend upon Company business objectives and business model. SOPs are Level 2 quality documents and, along with other relevant quality documents, ensure the effectiveness and efficiency of quality systems.

The ICH GCP guideline defines SOPs as "detailed, written instructions to achieve uniformity of the performance of a specific function". Simply put, SOPs specify in writing, who does what and when, or the way to carry out an activity or a process. SOPs establish a systematic way of doing work and ensure that work is done consistently by all persons who are required to do the same task. SOPs must be well written in order to provide an effective control of GCP and prevent errors from occurring, thereby minimizing waste and rework.

To be user friendly, they should be clear, unambiguous and must be written in plain language. SOPs are controlled documents and are best written by persons involved in the activity, process or function that is required to be specified or covered in the SOP. SOPs must be reviewed prior to their approval for release, for adequacy, completeness and compliance with company standards and all applicable legal, ethical and regulatory requirements. They must be reviewed and updated as required over their life cycle and any changes made to the SOPs must be re-approved. They must bear a revision status on them and their distribution must always be documented and controlled. When obsolete SOPs are required to be retained for any purpose, they should be suitably identified to prevent unintended use.

SOPs are mandatory for the implementation of GCP and other GxPs, namely, cGMP and GLP, within the scope of quality systems; therefore, it is well said that without SOPs there are no GxPs: no SOPs and no quality systems.

For an activity to become the topic of an SOP, it must be either subject to regulations or it must address a task important within quality systems or between quality systems and other functional units.

Quality systems related SOPs should generally cover the following topics in order to capture the core quality control and quality assurance activities and processes:

- Definition, format, content, review, approval, update, distribution and archiving of quality management plan;

- Definition of and activities related to quality control of clinical trials and compilation of trial-specific quality control plan;

- Initiation and maintenance of personnel files including format and content of curriculum vitae, job description, training records and personal and professional development plan;

- Top management reviews of quality systems and issuance of management review reports;
- Selection and management of contract auditors;
- Format, content, compilation, review, approval, update, distribution and archiving of audit program;
- Format, content, compilation, review, approval, update, distribution and archiving of audit plan
- Planning, conduct, reporting and close-out of riskbased internal and external audits;
- Planning, conduct, reporting and close-out of specific audits of sites, processes, systems and documents: sponsor site, third party (CRO, central clinical laboratory) site, investigator site, quality management system including SOP management, education and training and auditing, document management system including archives, data management system including information technology support, serious adverse events management system, pharmacovigilance system, medical dictionary management system, and regulatory submission documents (clinical trial reports, and clinical sections of new drug applications, marketing authorization applications, and common technical documents)
- Planning, conduct, reporting and close-out of for cause/directed audits;
- Hosting of customer audits;
- Preparation of sites for regulatory inspections;
- Coordination and management of regulatory inspections;
- Format, content, compilation, review, approval, update, distribution and archiving of CAPA plan, and assessment of its effectiveness;
- Change control to ensure that changes and the current status of quality systems related components including documents are identified; and
- Roles and responsibilities of quality assurance in handling of scientific misconduct/fraud.

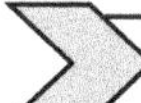 **Benefits of Quality Systems**

The importance of properly established and managed quality control and quality assurance systems with their integral well-written SOPs and other quality documents for the achievement of Company business objectives cannot be ignored. They serve as a passport to success by assisting the Company to achieve high-quality processes, procedures, systems, and people, with eventual high-quality products and services and enhancement of the following:

- Customer satisfaction, and therefore, customer loyalty and repeat business and referral;

- Timely registration of drugs by eliminating waste and the need for rework;
- Operational results such as revenue, profitability, market share and export opportunities;
- Alignment of processes with achievement of better results;
- Understanding and motivation of employees toward the Company quality policy and business objectives, as well as participation in continual quality improvement initiatives; and
- Confidence of interested parties in the effectiveness and efficiency of the Company as demonstrated by the financial and social gains from Company performance and reputation.

Table 5.1 Benefits of SOP

Benefit	Explanation
To provide people with all the safety, health, environmental and functional information necessitated to perform a job properly.	Placing value only on production while disregarding safety, health and environment is costly finally. It is better to train employees in all aspects of doing a job than to face accidents, fines and litigation later
To guarantee that production operations are performed constantly to obtain quality control of processes and products.	Consumers, from individuals to companies, want products of consistent quality and specifications. SOPs specify job steps that help standardize products and consequently quality.
To guarantee that processes continue uninterrupted and are completed on a prescribed schedule.	By following SOPs, you help to guarantee against process shut-downs caused by equipment failure or other facility damage
To guarantee that no failures occur in manufacturing and other processes that would harm anyone in the surrounding community.	Following health and environmental steps in SOPs guarantees against spills and emissions that threaten plant neighbors and create community outrage
To guarantee that acknowledged procedures are followed in compliance with company and government regulations.	Well-written SOPs help to guarantee that government regulations are satisfied. They also show a company's good-faith intention to operate perfectly. Failure to write and use good SOPs only signals government regulators that your company is not serious about compliance.
To serve as a training document for teaching users about the process for which the SOP was written.	Thorough SOPs can be used as the basis for supplying standardized training for employees who are new to a particular job and for those who need re-training.
To serve as a checklist for co-workers who observe job performance to reinforce proper performance.	The process of actively caring about fellow workers involves one worker coaching another in all aspects of proper job performance. When the proper procedures are outlined in a good SOP, any co-worker can coach another to help improve work skills.

Table 5.1 *Contd....*

Benefit	Explanation
To serve as a checklist for auditors.	Auditing job performance is a process similar to observation mentioned in the previous item only it usually involves record keeping. SOPs should serve as a strong basis when detailed audit checklists are developed.
To serve as an historical record of the how, why and when of steps in an existing process so there is a factual basis for revising those steps when a process or equipment are changed.	As people move from job to job inside and between companies, unwritten knowledge and skills disappear from the workplace. Regularly maintained written SOPs can chronicle the best knowledge that can serve new workers when older ones move on.

Writing style of SOP'S

SOP should be written in a step-by step, easy to read format by subject matter experts who know the process and the structure of the organization. They should be written by individuals aware of the activity and the organization's internal structure.

When it comes to writing effective SOP'S in pharmaceuticals, there are a few important things to keep in mind. First and formost, make sure your SOP's are concise and easy to understand.

It is very necessary to update SOP's as necessary to reflect changes in your industry or technology.

Keep your SOP's concise and easy to understand.

One of the key factors in ensuring effective SOP''s is making them concise and easy to understand. This will ensure that everyone involved in company's operation is aware of them and easy to follow them easily. These SOPs are divided into:

- Raw Materials
- Biological Products
- Facility
- Equipment (production & QC)
- Production
- Packaging
- Quality Control
- Quality Assurance

Here is a list of all the SOP's that is important for a pharmaceutical quality assurance.

List of all SOPs Related to Quality Assurance:

SOP for preparation of SOP

SOP for data integrity

SOP for in house code and numbers

SOP for document control, approval, revision, and authorization

SOP for market complains for market recalls

SOP for market returns and expiration goods

SOP for recovery from rejections

SOP for status labeling, color coding in premises

SOP for housekeeping audits

SOP for internal quality audits

SOP for checking, storage, and destruction of BMR/BPR and other production recodes

SOP for storage condition for finished goods

SOP for line clearance

SOP for total IPQA

SOP for process validation

SOP for cleaning method validation

SOP for testing method validation

SOP for purified water loop validation

SOP for batch control recores

SOP for QA documentation

SOP for equipments/machine qualifications

SOP for approval of batch coding and overprinting on packing materials

SOP for stereo order, receipt, checking, and issue

SOP for the disposal of expired printed packing materials

SOP for deviation reports

SOP for operation cleaning, calibrations, and maintenance of all machines and equipment

SOP for investigation out of specifications (OOS)

SOP for OOT (Out of Trending)

SOP for root cause analysis

SOP for change control

SOP for risk analysis, measurement, and controls.

SOP for review of BMR and BPR

SOP for good documentation practices

SOP for specimen signature

SOP for preparation, approval and execution of validation protocols and reports

SOP for validation master plans preparation, approval & review

SOP for FMEA (Failure mode & Effective Analysis)

SOP on handling and investigations of noconformances

SOP for inprocess checking

SOP for inpection and release of final goods

SOP on technology Transfer

SOP for failure investigation

SOP for power failure

SOP for Acceptance Quality Level (AQL)

SOP for operation of the data logger, monitoring of temperature and RH and evaluation of recorded data

SOP for handling of product yield

SOP for reconciliation of primary and secoundary packing material

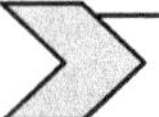

SOP General Format

SOPs should be organized to ensure ease and efficiency in use and to be specific to the organization which develops it. There is no one "correct" format; and internal formatting will vary with each organization and with the type of SOP being written. Where possible break the information into a series of logical steps to avoid a long list.

The level of detail provided in the SOP may differ based on, e.g., whether the process is critical, the frequency of that procedure being followed, the number of people who will use the SOP, and where training is not routinely available. A generalized format is discussed next.

Title Page

The first page or cover page of each SOP should contain the following information: a title that clearly identifies the activity or procedure, an SOP identification (ID) number, date of issue and/or revision, the name of the applicable agency, division, and/or branch to which this SOP applies, and the signatures and signature dates of those individuals who prepared and approved the SOP. Electronic signatures are acceptable for SOPs maintained on a computerized database.

Table of Contents

A Table of Contents may be needed for quick reference, especially if the SOP is long, for locating information and to denote changes or revisions made only to certain sections of an SOP.

Text

Well-written SOPs should first briefly describe the purpose of the work or process, including any regulatory information or standards that are appropriate to the SOP process, and the scope to indicate what is covered. Define any specialized or unusual terms either in a separate definition section or in the appropriate discussion section. Denote what sequential procedures should be followed, divided into significant sections; e.g., possible interferences, equipment needed, personnel qualifications, and safety considerations (preferably listed in bold to capture the attention of the user).

Finally, describe next all appropriate QA and quality control (QC) activities for that procedure, and list any cited or significant references. As noted above, SOPs should be clearly worded so as to be readily understandable by a person knowledgeable with the general concept of the procedure, and the procedures should be written in a format that clearly describes the steps in order.

Use of diagrams and flow charts help to break up long sections of text and to briefly summarize a series of steps for the reader. Attach any appropriate information, e.g., an SOP may reference other SOPs. In such a case, the following should be included:

1. Cite the other SOP and attach a copy, or reference where it may be easily located.

2. If the referenced SOP is not to be followed exactly, the required modification should be specified in the SOP at the section where the other SOP is cited.

TYPES OF SOPs

SOP's may be written for any repetitive technical activity, as well as for any administrative or functional programmatic procedure, that is being followed within an organization. General guidance for preparing both technical and administrative SOPs follows.

Guidelines for Technical SOP Text

Technical SOPs can be written for a wide variety of activities. Examples are SOPs instructing the user how to perform a specific analytical method to be followed in the laboratory or field (such as field testing using an immunoassay kit), or how to collect a sample in order to preserve the sample integrity and representativeness (such as collection of samples for future analysis of volatile organic compounds or trace metals), or how to conduct a bioassessment of a freshwater site.

Technical SOPs are also needed to cover activities such as data processing and evaluation (including verification and validation), modeling, risk assessment, and auditing of equipment operation. Citing published methods in SOPs is not always acceptable, because cited published methods may not contain pertinent information for conducting the procedure-in-house.

Technical SOPs need to include the specific steps aimed at initiating, coordinating, and recording and/or reporting the results of the activity, and should be tailored only to that activity. Technical SOPs should fit within the framework presented here, but this format can be modified, reduced, or expanded as require.

Title Page

Procedures - The following are topics that may be appropriate for inclusion in technical SOPs. Not all will apply to every procedure or work process being detailed.

(a) Scope and Applicability (describing the purpose of the process or procedure and any organization or regulatory requirements, as well as any limits to the use of the procedure),

(b) Summary of Method (briefly summarizing the procedure)

(c) Definitions (identifying any acronyms, abbreviations, or specialized terms used),

(d) Health & Safety Warnings (indicating operations that could result in personal injury or loss of life and explaining what will happen if the procedure is not followed or is followed incorrectly; listed here and at the critical steps in the procedure),

(e) Cautions (indicating activities that could result in equipment damage, degradation of sample, or possible invalidation of results; listed here and at the critical steps in the procedure),

(f) Interferences (describing any component of the process that may interfere with the accuracy of the final product),

(g) Personnel Qualifications/Responsibilities (denoting the minimal experience the user should have to complete the task satisfactorily, and citing any applicable requirements, like certification or "inherently governmental function"),

(h) Equipment and Supplies (listing and specifying, where necessary, equipment, materials, reagents, chemical standards, and biological specimens),

(i) Procedure (identifying all pertinent steps, in order, and the materials needed to accomplish the procedure such as:

- Instrument or Method Calibration and Standardization
- Sample Collection
- Sample Handling and Preservation
- Sample Preparation and Analysis (such as extraction, digestion, analysis, identification, and counting procedures)
- Troubleshooting
- Data Acquisition, Calculations & Data Reduction Requirements (such as listing any mathematical steps to be followed)
- Computer Hardware & Software (used to store field sampling records, manipulate analytical results, and/or report data)

(j) Data and Records Management (e.g., identifying any calculations to be performed, forms to be used, reports to be written, and data and record storage information).

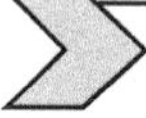 **Quality Control and Quality Assurance Section –**

QC activities are designed to allow self-verification of the quality and consistency of the work. Describe the preparation of appropriate QC procedures (self-checks, such as calibrations, recounting, reidentification) and QC material (such as blanks - rinsate, trip, field, or method; replicates; splits; spikes; and performance evaluation samples) that are required to demonstrate successful performance of the method.

Reference Section - Documents or procedures that interface with the SOP should be fully referenced (including version), such as related SOPs, published literature, or methods manuals. Citations cannot substitute for the description of the method being followed in the organization.

This can be well illustrated with the help of an example.

Example 1:

STANDARD OPERATING PROCEDURE		SOP No.	HSS/ZZZZ-NNN
		Effective Date	**xxxx**
Department	Quality Assurance	**Supersedes**	Nil
Title	Determination of CQA's/CMA's/KPP's/CPP's and Packaging parameters	Page No	Page 82 of 21

Purpose:

For identification of CMA, CPP, CQA & Packaging Parameters to lay down the procedure for drug products manufactured at pharmaceutical company.

Scope:

This SOP is applicable to manufacturing locations of pharmaceutical company for intended purpose. Continued Process Verification applicable for both new product and legacy product.

Responsibility:

Designated QA Person:

To prepare determination of CQA's/CMA's/KPP's/CPP's/Packaging parameters for legacy product.

To compile and review the data of continued process verification activity.

Head – Site QA/Designee:

To review determination of CQA's/CMA's/KPP's/CPP's/Packaging parameters for legacy product.

To ensure continuous monitoring of data and approve the continued process verification data.

Head – Production/Designee:

To review determination of CQA's/CMA's/KPP's/CPP's/Packaging parameters.

To investigate if any out of trend observed for commercialized drug products.

Head – Quality Control/Designee:

To investigate if any out of trend observed for commercialized drug products.

Head - PDL/Designee:

To review determination of CQA's/CMA's/KPP's/CPP's/Packaging parameters for Continued Process Verification.

Head – Quality/ Designee:

To approve determination of CQA's/CMA's/KPP's/CPP's/Packaging parameters for Continuous Process Verification.

To ensure this SOP is implemented at location.

Definition:

Continued Process Verification: Assuring that during routine production the process remains in a state of control.

Capability of a process: Ability of a process to produce a product that will fulfil the requirements of that product. The concept of process capability can also be defined in statistical terms.

Critical process parameter (CPP): A process parameter whose variability has an impact on a critical quality attribute and therefore should be monitored or controlled to ensure the process produces the desired quality.

Critical Quality Attribute (CQA): A physical, chemical, biological or microbiological property or characteristic that should be within an approved limit, range or distribution to ensure the desired product quality.

Critical Material Attribute (CMA): A material attribute whose variability has an impact on a critical quality attribute of a product and therefore needs to be monitored or controlled to ensure the process produces the desired quality of product.

EHS Requirement

NA

Procedure

Identification of CQA's, CMA's (API and Excipients), KPP's/CPP's and packaging parameters

In case of new drug products, CQA's, CMA's (API and Excipients), KPP's/CPP's of drug product and packaging parameters shall be provided by PDL/R and D along with tech transfer dossier.

In case of new drug products, in Process Qualification report CPP and CQA evaluated during process qualification are summarised and same shall be monitored throughout the product life cycle for continual assurance that the process remains in a state of control (the validated state) during commercial manufacture.

In case of existing commercialized drug products, CQA's, CMA's (API and Excipients), KPP's/CPP's and packaging parameters are identified by quality assurance based on product and process knowledge and experience.

Identified CQA's, CMA's (API and Excipients), KPP's/CPP's and packaging parameters shall be checked by PDL and final report parameter shall be used for continue process verification.

Criticality of CQA's, CMA's (API and Excipients), KPP's/CPP's and packaging parameters shall be assessed as per Form I.

Based upon the assessment decision upon the CQA's, CMA's (API and Excipients), KPP's/CPP's and packaging parameters to be monitored during CPV shall be made.

Training

Trainer : Head/Designee - Quality Assurance

Trainee : Quality Assurance staff, Quality Control, Production (G Block)

Attachment

Forms		
Sequential no.	**Form No.**	**Form Title**
Form-I	XXX	Determination of CQA's/CMA's, KPP's/CPP's, Packaging parameters for Continued Process Verification
Form-II	XXX	Continuous Process Verification Report

Distribution:

Location Department ↓	Unit I	Unit II	Unit III	Unit IV	Unit V
Quality Assurance	✓				
Quality Control		✓	✓	✓	
Production		✓	✓	✓	
Warehouse					
Engineering					
EHS					
IT					
Human Resources					

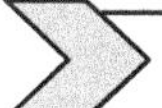 ## References & Linked Procedures

Reference:

PDA (Parenteral Drug Association), Technical Report No. 60, 2013

9.1.2 ISPE discussion paper PV stage 3, Process Validation: Applying CPV expectations to new and existing products.

Abbreviation

Abbreviation	Details
SOP	Standard Operating Procedure.
CPV	Continued Process Verification
CMA	Critical Material Attribute
CQA	Critical Quality Attribute
CPP	Critical Process Parameter
KPP	Key Performance Parameter

Contd....

Abbreviation	Details
Sr. No.	Serial Number
QA	Quality Assurance
QC	Quality control
SOP	Standard Operating Procedure
QA	Quality Assurance
R&D	Research and Development

Revision History

Revision No.	Change Control No.	Change Details	Reason For Change

As we can see that above example gives us a brief review of how in industry the SOP'S are designed and a entire department is responsible for the execution of the same. In short to summarize this statement we can say that SOP'S are tested, verified, approved, and documented way of executing operations that form the pharmaceutical industry's basis. It provides step-by-step guidance for the personnel to perform a specific process.

It is a Regulatory Requirement

Various standardization and regulatory bodies such as EU GMP and FDA require Standard Operating Procedures (SOPs) as a part of their regulatory requirements.

During their process inspection, they start by first reviewing the SOP for that particular process.

They inspect whether the process or procedure has its SOP and whether the process is executed according to the SOP. They can issue a warning or non-conformance if there is no SOP or there is a deviation between executed process and the approved SOP.

Ensures Consistent Results

SOPs are rigorously tested and verified for accuracy by relevant personnel.

If it passes acceptance criteria, only then are they implemented in the production process.

The SOP testing and verification activity help produce consistent results for every manufacturing process, batch or lot.

It also prevents deviations from standard results and helps prevent failure.

Unfortunately, in practice SOPs in the pharmaceutical industry are too often constructed and implemented for regulatory purposes only. As a result, they have been built for years as "houses to which one would add a room for each life event", gradually losing their overall coherence.

Each deviation (non-conformity / deviation from the standard process) is an opportunity to add a page, a paragraph or a sentence. As the years go by, the document becomes heavier and heavier, less and less usable for the operator who prefers to use his memory rather than to find the right information hidden in a document that is often unusable. The paper format is now outmoded by the digital tools available to the pharmaceutical industry.

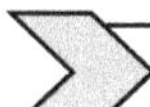

Important Questions

1. For which purpose manual SOP'S are required?

2. How do we ensure that SOP'S are followed?

3. How will you classify your process SOP'S?

4. Briefly describe the benefits of SOP.

5. It is very important to briefly write the SOP'S in a proper format. Explain.

6. Briefly describe the general format of SOP'S.

7. What are the Guidelines for Technical SOP Text?

8. With an example highlight how a SOP is designed?

9. How many types are the SOP?

10. How can you validate the SOP?

11. Who can prepared the SOP in Pharmaceutical Industry? and Explain the duty of SOP reviewer and implementer.

CHAPTER 6

Quality Defects – Achieving Zero Defects Policy

In treatment of diseases, Quality and safe medicines are required which would save the human lives. Pharmaceutical Industry is one of the sectors with most stringent guidelines since it deals with human lives. Defective products from this sector is least anticipated. Defective product is the one which couldn't fulfill the need of customer and may possess some degree of risk if it is used. If such product is released into the market, there are few consequences which manufacturing company would go through. Though Global Regulatory authorities, ICH and WHO have laid guidelines, we aren't successful in preventing even minor defects such as discrepancies in label specification. The objective of this chapter is to briefly discuss about the Pharmaceutical defects, Real-life product defects compared to textbooks recorded defects, their consequences and recent voluntary product recalls published by US-FDA which could help the Pharmaceutical Industry in enhancing their quality system.

As said by Johann Wolfgang, "Certain defects are necessary for the existence of individuality" but the same is not expected in pharmaceutical products. Pharmaceutical products are referred to be the golden sword for the treatment of ailments and any defects in them would cause a threat to precious human life. Cambridge dictionary defines a defect as "A fault or problem in something or someone that spoils that thing or person or causes it, him, or her not to work correctly". Pharmaceutical product defect holds a way different meaning since it is essential to save lives. Pharmaceutical product defect can be any change in the product that outweigh the drug's positive benefits.

To guarantee the quality of medicine, various measures are taken within the pharmaceutical industry. First, incoming goods are checked before they are used. During the subsequent production process, the following measures are taken: the production areas are set up following GMP standards, in-process controls are carried out during the production process, only validated equipment will be used, etc. After the entire production process, the batches are subjected to strict quality control.

Possible deviations from the process or questionable/OOS laboratory results are always closely examined and followed up. The final product is only released on the market when the QP, after verification of the different analysis results, gives certification of the batch. A watertight system one would think. However, it is still possible for a non-compliant product to make its way to the market despite the many measures we take to prevent it from doing so.

It's common for pharmaceutical startups and scale-ups to experience growing pains as they approach market approval. However, the best time to comply with current good manufacturing practices (cGMP) for quality isn't after you've failed an inspection, it's before you receive a warning.

Your ways of doing things may seem to work until an FDA inspector uncovers issues that have been overlooked, such as a batch of maintenance records that weren't reviewed the week your lab manager went on vacation.

Fortunately, there's an easier path than just hoping for the best when an FDA inspector arrives on site. One way to ensure that a 483 doesn't show up in your mailbox is by understanding what the most common compliance issues in the pharmaceutical industry are so that you can focus on those areas.

General Classification of Defects

Manufacturing defects: These are defects that arise during the production or negligence in the Quality assurance department. E.g. Packed Broken tablets in a batch of production

Design defects: this type may lead to defects in the entire line of manufacturing unless it is rectified. The manufactured product composition or the design differs from the intended specifications. E.g. Altered uniformity in dispersion of dispersible tablets

System failure defects: There are standard regulatory guidelines for each sector to be followed during the manufacture. This type of defect occurs when the manufacturing system fails to follow those guidelines. E.g. Contaminated dosage forms.

Types of Pharmaceutical Defects classified by the Regulatory authorities:

Minor: These are insignificant to the patients' health and product performance. Most of these defects may or may not be identified by the patient. E.g. Spelling mistake in Product information leaflet (PIL)

Major: The harm caused by this kind of defect is higher than minor. The customer can easily identify this type of defect. Major defects may affect the intended action of the product. E.g. Broken film coated sustained release tablets within intact blister

Critical: This type of defect is most serious than the above two. The products with critical defects are unfit to use and cause an adverse effect. This may cause liability to the company's reputation and the patient's health. E.g. Softened enteric coated tablets, improper sealing of vials.

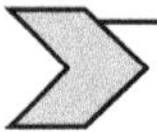

Comparison of Real-life Pharmaceutical Defects and Textbooks Recorded Defects

During the course of becoming a Pharmacy graduate our education system educates with all the knowledge to face the challenges in the Pharmaceutical Industry. The bitter truth is that real life is way different than the anticipated one. We would like to present an example for the above said lines.

Table 6.1

Dosage Form Type	Defects recorded	Real Life defects
Solid Dosage Forms		
Enteric coated tablets	Picking, Orange peel effect Lamination, Mottling, Blooming	Melted/Softened tablets in the blister
Uncoated tablets		Hair follicle inside intact blister
Film coated tablets		Dust formation inside tablet pocket with intact blister
Hard gelatin capsules	Weight variation, Contentuniformity, In vitro testing	Capsule sandwiched between foil and PVC film
Soft gelatin capsules		Dried soft gelatin capsules
Parenteral		
Dry powder parenteral	Visible particulate matter (Hair, Glass, Fibers) inside the ampoule or vial 10	Product on stopper

Table 6.1 Gives a comparison of Defects recorded in standard books and real-life defects which occur in the Pharmaceutical industry.

Every dosage form manufactured by the Pharmaceutical industry involves a number of unit operations which increases its vulnerability to be defective. But it is mandatory of time that defects shouldn't occur in medicines which are intended to save human lives. The Pharmaceutical Industry has to take all the necessary precautions and follow the regulatory guidelines.

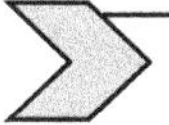 ## Consequences of Pharmaceutical Defects

Market complaints

When a market compliant is received it just implies that something is wrong with the sold product and customer is not satisfied. In Pharmaceutical industry market complaint indicates dissatisfaction regarding the clinical indication, quality or packaging which is lodged verbally or in written format.

Types of complaints:

1. Quality related: This category of complaints is related to physical, chemical or biological specifications or labelling and packaging condition of the product.
2. Adverse drug reactions related: Any noxious or unintended drug effects are reported by physician or patient to the Pharmacovigilance department.
3. Others: Lack of intended clinical efficiency or clinical response.

Fate of Market complaints

The journey of market complaint follows the Standard Operating Procedure (SOP) which is designed by the company. The complaint is received in customer complaint communication form with required details regarding the complaint.

QA head in coordination with QC head reviews documents such as analytical records, sampling and release records, and other raw data. Compliant is confirmed by QA head if there is significant difference in recorded values against the values of product in compliant. QA head checks for the stability data and if no issues are observed he shall process the compliant to Research and Development Head and QC head.

Once the inputs are received from respective departments QA head shall prepare summary of findings and shall share it in Customer compliant report format with customer and the management. Corrective and preventive actions have to be implemented to prevent any such incidents in future. The compliant is closed or in worst case scenario QA order for the product recall from the market. By coordination between supply chain and marketing department, marketed products can be recalled of that particular batch or lot

Drug recall or Product recall

It is a process of removal of products from the market that are not manufactured according to FDA's rules and regulation, to protect the public health from such defective products or It is a voluntary decision taken by the company or FDA's request to get back all the defective products which are in market manufactured by their company to prevent public from harmful products.

Drug recalls can also be classified based on who is initiating the product recall:

(a) *Voluntary or firm-initiated recall*: When the firm believes that the product released could impose risk to the public, it notifies the FDA to issue public notification.

(b) *Involuntary or FDA initiated recall*: This is initiated only during urgent situation where FDA monitors and coordinates with the recall procedure and strategy. Both type of recalls is subjected to legal action by FDA on the manufacturing firm. But a when the manufacturing firm takes the step of recall it has a huge impact on its customer's trust and would affect the customer's decision in buying their company drugs.

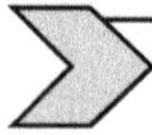 ## Recent Drug Product Recalls by USFDA

Due to lack of integrity in quality and safety of manufactured drug products, FDA is issuing product recalls order to number of companies whether they may be an innovator company or generic company.

Table 6.2 gives an overview of a few recent voluntary drug recalls published by US-FDA15. The observation made from the table is that all types of defects and product recalls are imposed even for products of reputed pharma companies and we aren't able to take necessary actions to prevent even the minor defects such as discrepancies in labelling.

Table 6.2 Recent voluntary drug recalls by reputed Pharma companies

Date	Generic name	Reason for recall	Company name	Class defect	Class of recall
04/15/2020	Nizatidine Oral Solution 15mg/mL	Presence of NDMA (NNitrosodimethyl mine)	Amneal Pharmaceuticals	Critical	I
04/13/2020	Hydromorphone HCL Injection, USP	Presence of empty and cracked vials	Hospira, Inc	Major	II
04/09/2020	Alka-Seltzar Plus	Discrepancies in primary label and secondary label	Bayer	Minor	III
03/26/2020	Phytonadione single dose ampoules USP, 10mg/mL	Inefficient strength of ampules resulting breakage	Dr. Reddy's Laboratories Ltd	Major	II
12/17/2019	Ranitidine tablets 150mg and 300mg	Presence o NDMA (N-Nitrosodi-methylamine)	Glenmark Pharmaceutical, Inc	Critical	I

To prevent the unforeseen defects and issues in manufacturing the Pharmaceutical manufacturers have to enhance their quality system. For Pharmaceutical Quality enhancement, ICH recommends to follow ICH Q10 guidelines which is comprehensive guideline of "Q8 Pharmaceutical Development and Q9 Quality risk management".

1. **Absence of written procedures or failure to follow written procedures**

   21 CFR 211.22(d) "The responsibilities and procedures applicable to the quality control unit are not in writing or fully followed."

   21 CFR 211.100(a) "There are no written procedures for production and process controls designed to assure that the drug products have the identity, strength, quality, and purity they purport or are represented to possess."

   In 2020–2021, the FDA issued 80 citations for procedures not in writing or fully followed and then gave out 44 citations for the absence of written procedures.

   Probably the most significant concern for anyone responsible for implementing, deploying, and maintaining a quality management system is effectively documenting procedures and work instructions that are easy to understand and execute.

   FDA CFR directs that pharma organizations must create written standard operating procedures (SOPs) for production and process control. These SOPs must include all requirements for drug identity, strength, quality, and purity. SOPs should be reviewed and approved by the operational and quality control units. Organizations must document compliance with these SOPs and create a record with clear justification any time operations deviate from the SOPs.

   In addition to noncompliance or issues of inadequate SOPs, analysis of 483 observations issued for CFR 211.100 in a recent year are often related to management and training. Excerpts from 483 letters have included the following language:

   Your firm has not established appropriate written procedures.

   There are documented instances of failure to follow SOP.

   Your firm's QC unit failed to approve procedures.

   SOP revisions are not documented appropriately.

   No records of cGMP training specific to SOPs.

   Both the GM and the Production Supervisor stated that they were unaware of [the SOP].

   Your SOP [is] in English. However, one operator ... cannot read English.

   Many of these issues can be corrected with better transparency and workflows. An electronic QMS for pharmaceutical companies can enable the QC unit and production leads to collaborate more effectively throughout the approval and revision process and ensure all necessary records are updated.

Common SOP pitfalls

Clear SOPs aren't just a regulatory requirement, however. Strong procedures are a roadmap for quality. Consistent procedures lower noncompliance, deviations, and ineffective data—but common pitfalls can get in the way of this.

Not collaborating

SOPs should be living documents. Creating and maintaining these documents should be a collaborative effort between the QC unit, leadership, and employees. It's not enough to pull together a document at the QC unit level and route it for necessary signatures. Employees should feel empowered to provide feedback and communicate.

Unclear roles and responsibilities

SOPs can be deliberately vague without mentioning specific roles. A document may say "the laboratory is responsible for" instead of "the laboratory manager." Clearly defined roles and responsibilities make it easier for employees to comply with quality processes, and it helps the QC unit link training activities to procedures.

Difficult format or language

SOPs shouldn't be a long, rambling document written in technical language. They should be clear, step-by-step instructions that show employees exactly how to complete a task.

2. Failures in laboratory controls

21 CFR 211.160(b) "Laboratory controls do not include the establishment of scientifically sound and appropriate specifications, standards, sampling plans or test procedures designed to assure that components, drug product containers, closures, in-process materials, labeling or drug products conform to appropriate standards of identity, strength, quality, and purity."

Pharmaceutical companies received 40 citations for not having scientifically sound laboratory controls from October 2020 to September 2021. Scientifically sound laboratory controls provide accurate, trustworthy lab data. cGMP for sound lab controls include:

Scientifically sound and appropriate specifications, standards, and test procedures

Monitoring the reliability, accuracy, precision, and performance of test procedures and instruments

Identification and handling of test samples

An FDA laboratory inspection focuses on both lab operations and raw data to determine whether a pharma organization is compliant with cGMP. You can expect an inspector to look at:

Lab records and logs

SOPs

Analytical procedures

Raw lab data

Lab equipment

Scientifically sound lab procedures are an enormous responsibility. Procedures, raw data, and management records are all necessary evidence of quality-driven operations. Raw data can tell a story about compliance and management, including instrument calibration, employee adherence to SOPs, and management investigations to find the root cause of operations.

3. Faulty production record reviews

21 CFR 211.192

"There is a failure to thoroughly review any unexplained discrepancy or the failure of a batch or any of its components to meet any of its specifications, whether or not the batch has been already distributed."

There were 49 observations given between October 2020 and September 2021 to pharma companies that didn't meet standards for the investigation of discrepancies or failures. CFR dictates that the pharma QC unit must review and approve all drug production and control records, including packaging and labeling records, to determine compliance with SOPs. If there is a discrepancy or failure, the QC is responsible for performing a thorough investigation and creating a report that includes conclusions and follow-up actions.

A clearly defined workflow for review and investigations is crucial to ensure nothing is omitted. There are numerous ways organizations can become noncompliant with CFR 211.192, which include:

Failure to review all logs

Downtime logs, cleaning logs, and clearance logs should all be subject to review

Procedural failures

Laboratory workers cannot review their own work or batch records

Lack of shared procedures

The QC unit and operations team should have a unified set of standards and SOP for batch record review to ensure there isn't any confusion around parameters.

4. Improper cleaning / sanitizing / maintenance

21 CFR 211.67(a) "Equipment and utensils are not cleaned, maintained, or sanitized at appropriate intervals to prevent malfunctions or contamination that would alter the safety, identity, strength, quality, or purity of the drug product."

The FDA issued 33 observations to pharmaceutical companies for not complying with 21 CFR 211.67(a), which is almost 3% of the letters that were sent between October 2020 and September 2021.

FDA CFR dictates that equipment and utensils are sanitized, maintained, and cleaned appropriately to prevent malfunctions or contamination. In other words, if your company is making medicine, then the FDA wants to ensure that you're working in a clean, sanitized environment.

SOPs should be followed for cleaning and maintenance, including:

- Responsibility for cleaning

- Maintenance and cleaning schedules

- Detailed work instructions of methods

- Protecting clean equipment from contamination

- Inspecting equipment for cleaning before use

- Maintaining records of maintenance, cleaning, sanitizing, and inspection

Analysis of 483 observations for 21 CFR 211.67(a) in one recent year revealed the following reasons for noncompliance at pharmaceutical organizations:

Maintenance activities have been performed "as needed" and logged on loose paper.

Forty-three of approximately 55 maintenance records weren't signed by the responsible employee.

Cleaning records were not reviewed and approved after tasks were performed.

SOPs failed to instruct technicians to record data for each maintenance activity.

Many 483 observations within this category result from visible maintenance or cleaning issues. Observations have cited equipment that is out-of-order or issues such as holes in a laboratory ceiling or rust that could compromise a clean environment. However, many result from improper procedures and aren't necessarily the result of a dirty lab. Frequent review of SOPs is necessary to ensure there are written procedures to protect drug quality and avoid contamination. Clear workflows in an e QMS can prevent the risk of activities that aren't reviewed or appropriately approved in compliance with cGMP.

5. Computer control of Master Formula Records

21 CFR 211.68(b)

"Appropriate controls shall be exercised over computer or related systems to assure that changes in master production and control records or other records are instituted only by authorized personnel."

If a company doesn't have certain documents stored properly where anyone can access them and edit them, they could get a 483 letter as a result. From October 2020 to September 2021, the FDA sent out 30 violations for this. Pharmaceutical companies need to have some documents that are only available to leadership and other key stakeholders to edit or approve edits to maintain the integrity of those files. Documents that need to be protected include anything related to drug development, data on clinical trials, and anything related to product quality.

When documents aren't protected from unauthorized edits, your critical records can potentially be compromised. Setting up track changes and approvals for edits within quality management system software can help prevent that and give companies a chance to stay compliant with this regulation. Plus, the software can easily display who changed what and when, showing clear audit trails for when the FDA comes to visit.

Other potential issues that could cause a 483 letter include:

Input/output verification: 21 CFR 211.68(b) says that the degree and frequency of this are based on the "complexity and reliability of the computer or related system."

Failing to backup data: The FDA regulates that a backup file should be maintained, except in certain cases where processes use automation. In that case, you'll need a written record and validation data.

Steering clear of pharmaceutical compliance issues

No pharmaceutical company wants its first interaction with an FDA inspector to result in a 483 letter. While organizations who receive a 483 can correct non-compliance issues, receiving an FDA letter is a sign that your organization has overlooked important quality processes. The costs of quality and operational issues which go uncorrected are much higher long-term than the costs of continually complying with FDA best practices.

Compliance issues in life sciences rarely result from willful rebellion against cGMP. Most commonly, organizations receive a 483 observation because something was overlooked. Perhaps the lab manager forgot to review maintenance records after a week on vacation. Maybe lab employees lost the updated SOP and have been using an older copy at the point-of-work. Noncompliance issues are the result of broken workflows, collaboration, and simple human error. Fortunately, you can avoid many of these common issues with better visibility and a QMS that supports quality-driven operations.

Zero Defect – A Competitive Advantage

With the recent focus on producing high quality, affordable medicines, the pharmaceutical industry faces pressure to reduce expenses without compromising quality in manufacturing. Quality programs, such as Zero Defect, add value by reducing costs, significantly improving quality and making a predictable supply of medicines available to patients. One area in a pharmaceutical company where this concept can be immediately applied to great benefit is working with raw materials and components (raw materials).

Zero Defect is not a new term in the quality world; it was coined by **Philip Crosby** in his 1979 book entitled, *Quality is Free,* and has emerged as a popular, highly regarded concept in quality management. Zero Defect can provide an aspiration for the company to stay competitive.

Zero Defect is a process of continuously evaluating and improving end-to-end processes from the supplier to the company. The objective is to produce the highest quality product while reducing defects to the lowest possible level by using high-quality raw materials. Zero Defect is not a quick fix; rather, it is a collaboration between the company and its suppliers to improve processes.

The challenge for companies is to bring defect-free new products to patients faster and more inexpensively than ever. This has led them to evaluate their internal processes and operating models to find ways to reduce waste by focusing on reducing defects, quality issues in manufacturing and scrap and complaints, and by eliminating avoidable testing, while proactively adopting quality programs. Strong relationships between the company and its suppliers are essential for improving quality in the long run.

The Context

Some of the quality dimensions in this chapter can be used as strategic analysis and performance management tools that assist in moving a company closer to its continuous improvement aspiration. In this case, right-first-time (RFT) metrics for all raw-materials quality defects were analyzed for a period of 10 years to determine suppliers' performance. In addition, the reduction of recurring quality defects was analyzed as a measure of raw material quality improvement over a period of 5 years. Note that these two performance measurements are inversely proportionate and that RFT and recurring defects stabilized at 99.6% and 6 defects.

Although difficult to measure, the issue of quality due to raw materials may also be seen at manufacturing sites, leading to disruption in the manufacture of products and potential stock-outs. Hence, collaborating with internal stakeholders also provides opportunities to improve raw material handling and testing processes.

The Why

Most companies take reactive measures to reduce raw material defects, given the time constraints they are under and their general focus on fixing the issues to release products to the market for patients. Instead, companies should proactively identify, evaluate and prevent potential raw material defects. The proactive approach will help the company move from a "cost-driven" to "value-driven" mindset.

For raw material defect reduction, it is essential to have continuous improvement as the objective by increasing the understanding and capabilities of raw material suppliers. As part of the process, it is also important to continue evaluating and optimizing raw material supplier performance by reducing defects. Having a clear objective and taking such measures will unequivocally reduce waste, minimize the cost of quality, and provide a planned, predictable supply of high-quality medicines to the patients.

The What

To evaluate a company's readiness, all stakeholders must agree on a common definition of Zero Defect.

A company's objective should be to reduce defects in raw materials delivered by suppliers, ensuring that all lots of materials received from all suppliers meet the agreed-upon specifications/requirements.

Striving for Six Sigma performance for critical material attributes (CMAs) by effectively eliminating known defects and preventing potential defects leads to maintaining the highest product quality. While perfection may not be achievable, the quest for it will push quality and improvements to the point that is acceptable under even the most stringent metrics.

Our recommended definition of Zero Defect is the absence of any defects from the suppliers of raw materials, that is:

Raw materials lots received from the supplier are within the agreed-upon specifications/requirements

All quality attributes, as listed in specifications, are within and/or below the acceptance criteria (e.g., AQLs, ppm).

The How

Having a cross-functional team brainstorm to collect ideas about how to reach the goal of Zero Defect is a best practice.

The six areas of improvement, represent quality risk management and potential improvement opportunities for a company. An engrained quality mindset and prioritization principles should also be applied. In addition, considering the cultures of both the company and the supplier is important to the success of such an endeavor. The focus should remain on the critical raw materials.

Prioritization: Use the company's product portfolio to identify strategic raw material suppliers and prioritize the suppliers by the criticality of the raw materials supplied.

Usage and Handling: Ensure processes are in place at the company for proper handling of raw materials and are in alignment with the supplier's recommendation.

Use of Correct Tools: Ensure that the use of correct measuring tools and test methods at the company are in alignment with the supplier's recommendations.

Alignment of Specifications: Align on specifications of raw materials with the supplier, including agreed-upon CMAs.

Redefining the Receipt Inspection: Ensure that testing and inspection are in alignment with the supplier's recommendations.

Continuous Improvement Mindset: Educate suppliers about the company's raw material requirements and clearly define expectations.

A company should take a deeper dive into the data and prioritize critical materials supplied for strategic products, and then select suppliers based on the historical data of their performance, including defects and defect trends.

For Zero Defect to be successful, several enabling factors play an important role:

Prioritization: Stay focused on prioritization of raw materials and suppliers for strategic products.

Messaging: Ensure transparent communications to all levels of the company by simple messaging to build allies.

Visible Management Commitment: Ensure top management shows support for Zero Defect and encourages middle management to carry out the message.

Governance: Establish governance between the company and the suppliers to maximize commitment.

Sponsors: Consider having sponsors at the company and at the supplier who have a strong understanding of the raw materials for resolving escalation of disagreements and removing roadblocks.

Expertise: Engage and empower Six-Sigma experts who fully understand the issues, processes and impact on a company's products to help carry out raw material improvement.

Link to Supplier Quality Strategy: Relate reducing defects and decreasing internal customer pain directly to the company's overall supplier quality strategy.

The Problem

Company X was working with a packaging component supplier whose packaging components failed significant dimensional and visual inspections. In addition, the specifications, the inspection and test methods, and the defect criterion had been misinterpreted between the company and its supplier.

Consequently, Company X began examining alternatives using the Zero-Defect initiative for primary packaging raw material suppliers by applying the Define, Measure, Analyze, Improve, and Control (DMAIC) process. The emphasis on defining, measuring and analysis ensured that opportunities for improvement would be executed in a way that provided the most positive impact.

The Process

Company X first **defined** the project:

Developed a business case and project charter to clearly define expectations of both the internal team and the supplier team

Selected a project sponsor who was impacted the most

Selected project core team members

Limited the team size, adding ad hoc team members as needed

Mapped the project timeline

Established a communication plan

Updated the project charter and timelines as needed

The Company then determined how it would measure the processes and progress made:

Performed a GEMBA walk for process visualization

Developed a process flow and reviewed the end-to-end processes for

Manufacturing

Quality – inspection and testing

Shipping – both the internal material flow and supplier chain processes

Performed deviation and product-complaint analysis

Reviewed risk assessments and identified critical quality attributes

Classified defects as critical, major or minor using risk-scoring methods

Company X **analyzed** the data collected on:

Agreed-upon specifications for raw materials – inspection and test methods, inspection set-up aligned with USP <790> and a measurement system analysis

Critical quality attributes

Sampling strategy – outgoing for the supplier and incoming inspection for Company X

Raw material shipping process against the agreed-upon requirements

Supplier's Zero-Defect program and how it aligned with its customer service program

Based on the information gathered, Company X determined elements that could be **improved**:

Defined an implementation plan based on the findings from its analysis

Implemented corrective and preventive actions (CAPA)

Reviewed and monitored the improvement activities

Performed a CAPA effectiveness check

Adjusted the project timeline as needed

To ascertain that all systems were in **control**, Company X:

Performed efficacy monitoring of the incoming material for 12 months

Recognized that the number of defects had been reduced significantly, demonstrating that the preventive measures the supplier had implemented were highly effective

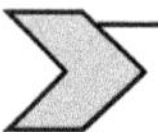

Conclusion

The management review process is the most important one since it monitors the functioning of other three elements. Management review process include observation of regulatory inspections and findings, enquiry on previous management reviews, training of personnel, improvements to manufacturing processes, confirmation of effectiveness of CAPA and most importantly measures which have been taken to minimize the customer complaints on product quality and product recalls from the market

Learning starts after the professional education from the University. None of us are aware of real-lifeproduct defects which could occur. The only measure which can be taken is learn from the past and implement required rules and regulation in the present to prevent any such defects in the future. Even though India being called as the Generic Capital of the World, several recalls have been initiated by Indian Pharma firms. The defects mentioned in this article may serve to alert the Pharmaceutical Industry to realize the type of defects which also could occur and take necessary measures to prevent them in future. To ensure the production of quality products each personnel from the stage of API manufacturing till the dosage form is placed into packaging material are responsible and required to stay alert thereby guarding the safety of patients and trust of customers in their company.

Pharma companies consider quality a strategic advantage and are aware of their quality niche. In order to stay competitive and uphold their reputations, they must remain focused on improving quality by exploring opportunities and pursuing quality measures in every aspect of production.

In summary, a focus on Zero Defect adds value to the product, significantly improves quality and provides a predictable supply of high-quality medicines to our patients. Continuing on this journey of effecting Zero Defect will support more patient benefits at less cost to society.

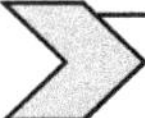 **Important Questions**

1. What are the factors affecting quality management system?

2. What are the factors affecting Quality management system?

3. What are the tools and techniques used during the Quality Planning process?

4. Briefly explain the general classification of Defects.

5. Enlist with examples the defects observed in Oral solid dosage forms.

6. Pharmaceutical defects can impose heavy consequences on pharmaceutical product. Explain/

7. Highlight different types of market complaints and its effect on end product.

8. What is Product recall? Explain with examples.

CHAPTER 7

Handling of Market Complaints and Recalls, Review of FDA-483 Form

The pharmaceutical industry introduces many therapies to the market; hence it is at an important place in medical innovations. If this industry stops working, many health problems would remain unsolved. Pharmaceutical industry can create several problems also due to topic called product complaint.

Product complaint is a topic of interest for all pharmaceutical industries, consumer health care companies, medical device manufacturer, and various other Industries governed by regulatory authorities. The product should be recalled from all the above, if complaints are found to be genuine.

Product complaints are, when any party or customer has reported any adverse event or product defect of any company's marketed product. The complaints can be from various sources like external or internal, or it can be verbal or written. If these complaints found to be genuine, the product should be recalled to the company.

The product recall is a procedure of retrieval or withdrawal of products known to be defective, promptly and effectively, from the market. As the pharmaceutical industry is one of the largest industry, generates enormous amount of sensitive and private information such as medical records, employee information, financial data and research data, it requires a effective Information Security Management.

Information Security Management is critical in the pharmaceutical industry and it can be a very big loss to the company to not having it.

Product complaint

Product complaint is either internal or external report regarding any product defect or dissatisfaction of customer. The internal complaint can be from warehouse, quality control, production and marketing division of the company. External complaint can be from doctors, clinics, hospitals, paramedics, pharmacies, drugstores, supermarkets, and customers. It can be of two forms like verbal or written like mail, letter, etc. The written complaints are received in writing. The verbal complaints are received by oral and must be documented by appointed person. In the pharmaceutical industry, handling of this product complaint is important issue because if there is a serious quality problem aroused, it can harm the customer, also to the company's reputation.

If product complaint received, it is necessary to identify and address the root cause of the complaint. Solution of root cause will help to prevent the recurring of complaints. Appropriately handled complaints can help to retain or get more customers and ensure customer satisfaction. If there are serious quality problems of product cause potential harm to the consumer, product recall shall be considered.

The handling of complaint will take a very important place in pharmaceutical industry, as this industry directly related to the human lives. The market product complaints should be handled in an appropriate manner. Procedure for handling of market complaints:

Introduction to Complaints

Complaints are indications of dissatisfaction with quality, performance or a defect after a drug product/ substance has been released for distribution. It is, therefore, an excellent post-market surveillance indicator.

A complaint could lead to rectifying/changing the manufacturer's systems. Complaints do not only refer to the drug product/substance, but also to its labelling and packaging. Complaints may or may not have significant impact on the health of the patient.

Complaints help in identifying product defects and possibly quality system problems, which might have not been adequately implemented in the company.

Handling of Market Complaints

Complaints may be received from various sources either verbally, in written form, or by electronic means, along with samples, photographs and/or other evidence depicting the defect. The source of complaints may be the patient, healthcare professionals, regulatory agencies, qualified pharmacists, trade sources, distribution chain personnel or any other source. Complaints are classified by the person handling complaints at the company after logging to prioritize the investigation.

Complaints can be classified into one of the follows:

- Critical
- Major
- Minor

Critical Complaints

Are those complaints about defects which impact the quality of the product and affect the patient. Examples of defects leading to critical complaints for drug products/drug substances can be listed as follows: product mix up, product not meeting regulatory specifications, contamination and microbial growth, presence of insect, mix up of printed packaging material, use of wrong printed packaging material, wrong labelling, serious adverse reactions leading to death, regulatory notices advising recall, failure to meet statutory labelling conditions, gross physical change in product (e.g., precipitation), wrong expiry date mentioned, missing dose of a critical therapeutic or life-saving drug, integrity breach, presence of metallic or glass contamination, etc.

Major Complaints

These are about defects that reduce the suitability of use of a dosage form for its intended purpose. Examples of complaints categorized as major complaints include oral dosage forms not meeting disintegration/dissolution norms, gross damage to packaging, serious ADE (expected), texture change, grittiness, contamination and microbial growth due to defective supply chain, etc.

Minor Complaints

These do not affect product quality. Such complaints relate mainly to defects that are cosmetic in nature. Some examples of such complaints are smudging of printed matter, shortage of tablets in a strip, broken tablets, missing blisters in cartons, missing leaflets or multiple copies of the same leaflet, etc.

Complaints can be further subdivided into substantiated and non-substantiated after the preliminary investigation is completed within three (03) days of logging the complaint.

Substantiated Complaints

Are those that are due to defects in process or systems employed by the manufacturing company. These complaints have sufficient evidence to support the suspicion of such defects.

Non-substantiated Complaints

These are those complaints which do not have sufficient evidence to support the suspicion of defect. These may not have occurred at all, or there is lack of evidence to prove the defect. These may occur due to improper handling of the drug product/substance. Use of the drug product in ways other than prescribed could also lead to misunderstanding by the patient resulting in such complaints.

There are other types of complaints also which could originate from therapeutic activity. They can be due to insufficient pharmacological activity, such as: Lack of Effect where the drug product is not able to effect sufficient pharmacological activity and reduce the discomfort of the patient. In many cases, such complaints could be the result of improper administration of the drug product by the patient.

Adverse Drug Reaction/Effect

These are events leading to unexpected reactions after administering a drug product, for example, the development of rashes, nausea, etc. Such events can take place in cases where combinations of two or more drugs are administered. Adverse drug reactions may occur for drug products administered for prolonged periods of time or even after a single administration.

Apart from all the above listed complaints, sometimes complaints lead to unexpected revelations. The defects reported may also result in identifying counterfeit samples. Counterfeit Complaints are those in which it has been proven that the defective product is a copy of the original product and does not belong to the manufacturing site printed on the label.

This can be proved only when the manufacturer receives samples of defective drug products from the complainant, and on matching these against the retained samples, differences are noticed. Regulatory agencies take complaints about drug products/substances very seriously and expect the manufacturer to respond in the shortest possible time.

There are several instances where the regulatory agencies follow up with the manufacturer and trigger unannounced inspections of facilities manufacturing products that are under the scanner. Systems, procedures and personnel involved in the process of manufacturing drug products/substances are required to follow robust practices where defects can be identified before the product/substance reaches the market.

Handling complaints is one of the most important functions of the manufacturing facility. Written procedures describing the handling of all complaints received through any mode regarding a drug product must be established and followed.

Such procedures could include provisions for review, by the site QA, of any complaint involving the possible failure of a drug product to meet any of its specifications and, for such drug products, a decision as to the need for an investigation in accordance with 21 CFR 211.192

Such procedures may include provisions for review to determine whether the complaint represents a serious and unexpected adverse drug experience which is required to be reported to the FDA in accordance with 21 CFR.

A written record of each complaint must be maintained in a file designated for drug product complaints. The file regarding such drug product complaints can be maintained at the establishment where the drug product involved was manufactured, processed, or packed; such a file may be maintained at another facility if the written records in such files are readily available for inspection at the facility from where the drug product in question originated.

Written records involving a drug product to be maintained for until at least one (01) year after the expiration date of the drug product, or for one (01) year after the date that the complaint was received, whichever is later. In the case of certain OTC drug products that do not need to provide for expiration dating because these meet the criteria for exemption under 21 CFR 211.137, such written records must be maintained for three (03) years after distribution of the drug product. The written record may include information such as name and strength of the drug product, lot number, name of complainant, nature of complaint, and reply to complainant.

If an investigation is conducted under 21 CFR 211.192, the written record can include the findings of the investigation and follow-up. The record or copy of the record of the investigation must be maintained at the establishment where the investigation occurred in accordance with 21 CFR 211.180(c).

If the investigation is not conducted under 21 CFR 211.192, the written record can include the reason that such an investigation was found not to be necessary together with the reason/s and the name of the responsible person making such a decision.

There are several instances of USFDA issuing 483's because of improper complaint handling. According to USFDA's 2016 enforcement statistics, product complaint handling system (21 CFR 211.198: Complaint Files) is the second most cited 483 with 326 EIR observations which was 3 % of overall EIR observations. of past 483's from USFDA reveal lack of inadequate procedures, failure to follow established procedures and lack of documented evidence (Good Documentation and Data Integrity) as primary causes of warning letters.

The complaint will receive by the marketing department or product promotion department and forward it to quality assurance department (QAD). The quality assurance department will file the complaint in register with reference number.

Handling of Complaints

This is the beginning of the investigation determining the authenticity of the complaint. This activity focuses on the detection of potentially defective drug products/substances. The QS/GMP regulation expects a set mechanism of review, evaluation and reporting once a complaint is received.

Trained professionals with authority to decide the outcome are expected to handle complaints. Handling complaints is one of the most important activities indicating willingness to resolve the dissatisfaction about the drug product/substance. Set procedures with timelines to address various stages involved in addressing complaints are expected by the regulatory agencies and are verified during their audits. Complaints trigger investigation to confirm the product's integrity and to prove the robustness of the manufacturing activity of the company.

Companies must have written procedures in place for processing complaints. Deficiencies in complaint handling procedures lead to losing valuable data which might help in identifying defective products and quality systems. Review mechanisms help- in identifying existing and/or potential causes of nonconforming product or other quality problems.

All competent authorities, concerned in the matter, including the complainant, must be informed in a timely manner in case the investigation leads to recall or abnormal restriction in the supply of the product if there is a confirmed quality defect like faulty manufacture, product deterioration, detection of falsification, non–compliance with marketing authorization, etc.

- Stages of handling complaints are as follows
- Receipt of complaint
- Categorization of complaint
- Notification to regulatory agency
- Initiating investigation
- Receipt and handling of samples
- Risk Assessment and CAPA
- Closure of the complaint
- Trending
- Historical review

Receipt of complaint

Site QA must receive the complaint.

Site QA must log the complaint within one (01) working day.

Complaint can be shared with PV if the nature includes ADR/ADE or a combination of these with product quality.

Complaint number must be assigned by site QA.

If the number of complaints is more than one (01) from the same complainant and for different products, different numbers shall be assigned for each complaint.

Site QA must acknowledge the receipt of complaint with the complainant within three (03) working days through the company's procedure.

Additional information, if required, with photographs and sample can be obtained from the complainant. Annexure ("Information from complainant") can be obtained from the complainant.

Categorization of the complaints

Site QA must categorize the complaint initially as critical or non- critical based on the nature of the complaint.

Site QA Head must confirm the categorization of the complaint.

Preliminary investigation

Preliminary investigation can be performed for critical complaints within three (03) working days from complaint awareness date.

Regulatory notification

Alert Notification/FAR can be filed by site QA with respective regulatory agency within three (03) working days from the complaint awareness date. The AN/FAR must include the preliminary investigation report.

Corporate Quality Head can be notified of the AN/FAR

All the batches/lots/markets likely to be impacted must be mentioned in the AN/FAR.

Follow-up reports and final AN/FAR can be filed along with the interim and final investigation reports respectively as per the commitment given in the initial AN/FAR.

Site QA Head must also report in a timely manner to the marketing authorization holder/sponsor and all competent authorities concerned in the matter about the detection of counterfeit, recall of the product or an abnormal restriction in the supply of the product.

Investigation

Complaints involving product quality can be investigated with cross-functional teams, wherever applicable, as per the investigation procedure of the company.

If the complaint is critical in nature, preliminary investigation must be completed within three (03) working days.

Investigation can be performed as per the investigation procedure of the company.

Investigation can be performed by adopting suitable tools like fishbone analysis/Ishikawa, 5-Whys analysis, brainstorming, etc.

Retention samples, complaint samples, input materials and any other samples as applicable will be subjected to investigation.

Batch records, in- process records, analytical records, stability data as applicable and all allied records must be reviewed as part of the investigation.

Historical review of product complaints/deviation/incident/investigations can be carried out to establish potential impact of market complaint on the concerned batch/other batches of same product/substance and/or other manufactured products.

Historical review of complaints from the previous two years (from the date of receipt of complaint) can be performed.

Additional experiments, if required, may be carried out with the help of relevant cross functional departments to establish the root cause of the defect as per approved study protocol.

Investigation of batches of the drug product/drug substance manufactured using the same raw material/key starting material/packing material of the complaint batch must be performed and if it leads to a possibly faulty equipment, the equipment may be subjected for investigation.

If preliminary investigation points to raw material(s), key starting material(s) and/or packing material(s) as likely cause of complaint, the balance stock material of the respective QC reference number used in the complaint batch can be quarantined till the completion of investigation.

Quarantine may be effective until clearance to use given by Site QA. Investigation can be extended to all batches of the same or other drug product/substance manufactured during the period in which the complaint batch was manufactured and impact assessment must be performed irrespective of whether the other batches were distributed or not.

Health Hazard Evaluation can be performed for the complaints covering the following, wherever applicable, but not limited to, product/strength mix-up, drug not available to the patient due to dissolution failure, degradation of product, etc.

Alert Notification/FAR can be communicated to the Regulatory Agencies within three (03) working days of detecting the defect irrespective of the stage of investigation. All customers must be notified about the defect within three (03) working days in case of drug substance.

The complaint/s due to counterfeiting can be assessed and if the sample is found to be counterfeit in nature, Marketing, QA/RA, and Regulatory Agencies in countries where the product is distributed must be informed for appropriate action.

Risk assessment can be carried out taking into account system failure during investigation. It could be performed as per QRM procedure. Risk Assessment for market complaints can be based on severity and occurrence.

The evaluation of risk to the quality of the drug product/substance can be assessed based on scientific knowledge and ultimately linking it to the patient's safety. Immediate actions may be taken to rectify the problem wherever applicable.

Appropriate CAPAs can be initiated based on the findings of the investigation and risk assessment. Site QA must implement the CAPA and monitor its effectiveness. Site Quality Assurance can assess whether the complaint is substantiated or non-substantiated and its impact on the marketed product.

Substantiated complaints can be categorised as Critical/Major/Minor based on the investigation findings by site Quality Assurance Head/Designate. Investigation must be completed in thirty (30) calendar days from complaint awareness date.

If investigation is incomplete within thirty (30) calendar days, an interim report must be prepared within the original due date and extension can be taken with justification. After completion of investigation, final investigation report must be prepared and shared with complainant.

Site Quality Assurance can initiate product recall, if applicable, based on the decision of recall committee as per recall procedure. Site Quality Assurance Head must notify Corporate Quality Head, all stake holders and management about the recall.

Receipt and handling of samples

Complaint samples must be photographed for depicting the nature of the complaint and labelled as "Complaint Sample" by site QA. The photographs must be attached along with the market complaint documents for future reference.

Three attempts can be made by site QA to collect the complaint sample and additional information for investigation if not received.

Investigation must be initiated based on available information. If the complaint sample is not available or submitted post follow-up within the timeline, the complaint can be closed. However, if the complaint sample is received after closure of the complaint, the same must be re-opened. The procedure of investigation and sharing information with stakeholders can be as per the procedure mentioned earlier.

All complaints received must be stored as per the prescribed conditions in designated area till closure of market complaints. Complaint samples may be retained for training purpose.

Site Quality Assurance Head/Designate can ensure the destruction of complaint sample after closure of the complaint.

Closure of complaint

Complaint must be closed by site QA in sixty (60) calendar days from complaint awareness date which includes the time period of thirty (30) calendar days for investigation.

In case where the investigation is extended beyond thirty (30) calendar days, the complaint can be closed after thirty (30) calendar days from the date of completion of investigation.

Site QA must ensure the initiation of action items for CAPA before the closure of the complaint.

Site QA can maintain the complaint records along with investigation records.

Trending of complaints

Trend analysis must be performed by Site Quality Assurance as per following steps:

- Identification of trending need
- Trending frequency
- Data collection and presentation
- Data verification
- Data Analysis
- Data evaluation and interpretation
- Trend analysis for product complaints must be based on product, dosage form, market, nature of complaint, categorization of complaint (initial and final category), substantiated/non-substantiated complaint, status of complaint (open/close), root cause, etc.
- Trend analysis for ADE complaints must be based on product, dosage form, market and category (seriousness and expectedness criteria).
- Frequency for trend analysis can be quarterly and annual.
- Trend analysis can be completed within one month of completion of quarter/year. Rolling data must be considered for trending.
- Trending data can be collected as per applicable QMS. Collected data must be compiled and presented by site Quality assurance.
- Data can be verified by cross functional team.
- The collected data must be analyzed by statistical/logical methods using appropriate tools like pie charts, bar charts, Pareto analysis, etc.
- Trending can identify KPIs which help in reduction or elimination of specific and repetitive defects.

- Trending can identify areas of improvement where there is any recurrence of problems.
- Appropriate CAPAs can be initiated accordingly.
- Impact of trend analysis must be considered for impact assessment on other products/batches.
- Summary report for trend analysis can be prepared by site QA and reviewed by the cross-functional teams and approved by site Quality Assurance Head.
- Under the supervision of quality assurance department head, the executive of quality assurance department will perform investigations by root caus.
- The maximum time for sending reply to customer should be of 15 days.
- All the complaints are reviewed yearly for evaluation of market complaints which are out of trends by annual review procedure.
- All the complaints related to quality, whether they received orally or in writing, they should be recorded and investigated according to the stated procedures.
- The complaint report should contain the following,
- Name and address of complainant
- Name and phone number of person submitting the complaint
- Complaint nature including name and batch number of the API
- Date at which complaint is received.
- Action initially taken including date and identity of person taking the action.
- Any follow up action taken
- Response provided to the complainant
- Final decision on intermediate or API batch or lot

Product recall

The product recall is a removal of marketed product from market for the reason of deficiencies in safety, quality and efficacy, including labeling considered being in violation of laws. For the effective management of product recall, it is important to know what the product recall constitutes of.

The decision to recall drug from market can be taken by the ministry of health, manufacturer, the licensee or the import permit holder. The reason of the recall of medicinal product can be any complaint from the customer or any unexpected and serious adverse drug reaction.

Any type of industry should have an efficient recalling system for fast removal of unsatisfactory material whenever the complaint arises. Once the decision of recall made, the responsibilities should be assign to separate personnel for implementation, this can help to achieve an efficient recalling system.

Every industry should have a product recall coordination committee to execute the recalls. The product recall co-ordination committee should constitute of:

- Managing director
- Quality assurance head
- Production head
- Marketing department head

The managing director will make the ultimate decision regarding recalls. A specific criterion should be followed by the manufacturer company for recall. When regulatory agency ordered, the recall co-ordination committee should recall the product.

Once complaint found to be genuine, the recall process must initiate within 48 hours and should be completed within 14 days. This product recall procedure should be done at different level, i.e., vendor, distributor, retailer, wholesaler, and user, by informing the supply chain. As soon as the product recalled from market, the recall co-ordination committee authorize a person to destroy the recalls at the site of manufacture.

The recalled product should be destroyed and documented in presence of the authorized personnel. A product recall usually results from one or combination of several situations like company discovery, customer complaint, adverse drug reaction, or regulatory inspection. In that, customer complaint can be any major and critical defect like stained labels due to leakage, precipitation in clear syrup, off odour.

The company discovery can include problems related to the running batch; a particular batch may have some problem during processing, the company carrying out an investigation might lead to the discovery of any problem with earlier batch which is not found prior to release can be included in company discovery e.g. change in viscosity.

Any adverse situation reported can also lead to the product recall. The product recall is classified into three types, class I, class II, and class III.

Class I recall includes reasonable probability that the exposure or use of violative product will cause serious adverse consequences or death. The class II recalls includes a situation in which the probability of serious adverse reactions can be controlled and exposure to violative product may cause temporary medically reversible adverse reaction. The class III includes a situation in which the exposure or use of violative product is not causing a adverse reaction.

The FDA-483

A *Focus* review (thanks to the Freedom of Information Act) of 50 Form 483s issued by the US Food and Drug Administration (FDA) to Indian pharmaceutical and active pharmaceutical ingredient (API) manufacturers over the past two years reveals a slew of detailed quality concerns from the agency.

And although the products described in the 483s have been redacted, and a majority of the FDA observations are for relatively commonplace documentation or procedural issues that will be (or already have been) corrected, there are a number of surprises, particularly as so many of the observations are for egregious errors like altering official documents in front of an inspector, or not maintaining bathrooms for employees, or documenting important manufacturing or electrical data on scrap paper in pencil.

What Is a 483?

Following an FDA inspection for a manufacturing plant – which usually lasts between three and seven days -- the agency provides a review of what it found, and based on that review, can issue a Form 483 to a company's management with observations of any conditions that in the inspector's judgement may constitute violations of the Food Drug and Cosmetic (FD&C) Act and related acts.

FDA investigators are trained to ensure that each observation noted on the FDA Form 483 is clear, specific and significant, though as this review of 483s reveals, no two 483s are alike, and even the forms provided to the companies vary.

FDA Presence in India

As the Indian generic drug and API industries continue to be one of the main suppliers to the US, FDA's presence in the country is important for ensuring the products are safe and effective. In February, FDA announced plans to double the number of its inspectors in India – from about nine to 19.

But even if FDA quadrupled its inspectorate in India, the agency would still have problems trying to physically inspect the more than 550 manufacturing sites the Indian government says are registered with FDA.

As far as the public release of Form 483s, FDA issues some of what it sends to foreign companies, though the vast majority of the reports have to be obtained via the Freedom of Information Act.

In addition to FDA, India's regulator, known as the Central Drugs Standard Control Organization (CDSCO), also inspects local and multinational companies' manufacturing facilities, although those inspection reports are not released publicly on its website and only one of the 50 Form 483s reviewed by *Focus* noted that CDSCO representatives were present for an inspection.

Recently, CDSCO announced it would set up a training program to address gaps in inspections. And CDSCO also has been uploading to its website a monthly list of drugs, devices and cosmetics that are either not of standard quality, spurious, adulterated or misbranded.

Companies Involved

All of the Indian companies receiving FDA Form 483s reviewed by *Focus* have products that are or were on the US market, though the sizes of the companies vary from small, like **Divis Laboratories**, to multi-national companies, like **Hospira, Dr. Reddy's** and **Wockhardt**, which has other manufacturing sites in the UK, Ireland, US and France.

Other companies receiving the 483s reviewed include: **Aarti, Akorn India, Ajanta Pharma, Agila Specialties, Apotex, Aurobindo, Cadila, Claris Injectables, Cipla, Emcure Pharmaceuticals, Glenmark Generics, Hetero, Indoco Remedies, Ipca Laboratories, Lupin, Mega Fine Pharma, Nosch Labs, Pan Drugs, Shlipa Medicare** and **Sri Krishna Pharmaceuticals.**

How Bad Does it Get?

Currently, 46 Indian manufacturing sites are listed on FDA's import alert list, which bars the sites from shipping products to the US. Some of the Form 483s reviewed by *Focus* deal with these restricted sites.

For instance, analysts working at **Aarti Drugs**, which has two facilities on the FDA import alert list, had directed company software to overwrite previously collected chromatography data, causing the originally collected result to be automatically deleted. FDA noted:

In addition, during FDA's review of batch manufacturing records at Aarti, inspectors found that manual manufacturing activities for two different products were performed at the same time by the same employee, which is physically impossible.

And during FDA's review of manufacturing operators' "Training Evaluation Papers," inspectors found that one quality assurance (QA) officer answered four of seven questions correctly during his evaluation following training on the company's "Deviation & Change Control" procedures, and the test was scored as "8/10" and considered satisfactory.

Similarly, at **Ipca Laboratories**, which is also on the import alert list, an inspector found that a quality affairs officer had partially shredded training validation forms for multiple manufacturing operators, though a quality affairs officers said it was a mistake.

Akorn India is another example of a company with a history of issues with FDA. The companyhas its Paonta Sahib site listed on the FDA import alert list, where FDA found during an inspection of the quality assurance validation office, the presence of unauthorized QA document control stamps and partially completed and/or unofficial training records for a significant number of manufacturing operators.

In addition, an environmental monitoring document, known as the "Microbial Air Sampling Report," was altered during the course of the firm's photocopying of the record for the agency.

"No explanation was provided regarding the reason for altering this cGMP document requested as a part of this inspection," FDA said.

For **Cadila Healthcare**, meanwhile, FDA found the company failed to adequately review 106 consumer complaints in 2013, and 132 in 2014.

FDA also apparently had to deal with a lack of willingness of the company to be forthcoming about incident reports. In one case, the inspector says: "After questioning more than five employees multiple times, the Vice President QA stated that the incident report is located offsite at an employee's home."

FDA also said this to Cadila concerning its recent recalls of products:

Data Quality

The issue of recording data properly from manufacturing operations is another one that continues to crop up in the Form 483s and elsewhere. Earlier this year, EMA recommended the suspension of a number of medicines that relied on clinical trials performed by **GVK Biosciences** that regulators were concerned had been manipulated.

In addition, over at **Apotex Research Private Limited,** which is dealing with other issues uncovered by Health Canada, FDA inspectors found that a QC microbiologist "was observed overwriting the dates for previously read (awaiting disposal) growth promotion plates using a black marker in order to make it appear that the growth promotion testing had been performed previously."

And during a review of the firm's analytical QC laboratories, FDA identified a company practice of retesting drug product samples when failing and/or otherwise undesirable chromatography results were encountered. FDA also had issues with the company's testing of drug samples.

The same issue cropped up at **Mylan Laboratories'** Bangalore facility, where FDA inspectors said the good manufacturing practice (GMP) records used to record activities occurring inside the filling rooms are laminated pages. "Original raw data is recorded in marker on the surface of the laminated sheets. The marker can be erased," FDA said, noting that there were examples where it appeared original data "had been erased and written over."

In a review of **Sun Pharmaceutical**'s site in Ahmednagar, India -- which is not the import alert list, though another company site in Karkhadi is -- FDA inspectors found in one of the manufacturing areas, scrap paper for what appeared to be multiple manufacturing batches' data, and while in the engineering electrical area, an inspector observed seven scrap papers which appeared to contain electrical raw data.

For another Sun site in Dadra, India, inspectors found that six "generic" user accounts had been created in the Laboratory Information Management software system, which are not traceable to the employee using the software, though users could delete particle size values, change sample weights, change related substance value entries and make other changes.

What's to Come?

Although a number of these companies will (or already have) received warning letters from FDA or been placed on the import alert list based on these initial inspections, it's difficult to gauge whether FDA has hit the tip of the iceberg with data integrity issues, or is seeing progress in how companies address them.

And because the inspections all deal with sensitive information, the best and only way to track these issues is to continue following the release of inspection reports from regulators worldwide, as well as the slow trickle of companies self-reporting when they receive a 483 or warning letter.

The FDA-483 is a form used by FDA investigators for inspection. It is required to officially record inspectional result at the completion of an investigation. The FDCA requires the written inspectional observations. Whenever an investigator found that the drug may be adulterated or is being packed, or processed under conditions which are not confirm to specification, then the 483 observations are made.

On the last day of inspection, these forms are presented to the management. A deadline is given by the FDA for submission of response within 15 days to the firms. The agency will not review the response before issuing a warning letter, if FDA received the response after 15 working days.

Some of the non-GMP areas post marketing issues related to adverse drug reaction are observed in the FDA-483. These are reported in the descending order of significance. It also contains the observations of some objectionable practices but is not listed on FDA-483; they are verbally discussed with the firms during the inspection and are reported in the establishment inspection report (EIR). This FDA-483 form does not contain observations related to the style of labeling, content of label, and promotional material, etc. Impact of a significant FDA-483

The FDA-483 forms gives impact on both import and export. In case of export, the FDA policy states that the certificate to foreign government (CFGs) will not give if the manufacturing facility for the product to be exported is not in compliance with the good manufacturing process.

In case of import, FDA can authorize refuse for the products that appear to be misbranded, adulterated, or unapproved without their physical examinations. The FDA has authority to issue import alerts for foreign manufacturing companies.

An **FDA 483** observation, or "inspectional observation," is a notice sent by the FDA to highlight any potential regulatory violations found during a routine inspection. This can relate to the company's facility, equipment, processes, controls, products, employee practices, or records.

An **FDA 483 observation can be very expensive**, resulting in thousands or even millions of dollars in costs for some companies. If the issues are systemic, the Form 483 observation can trigger training, redesign, process implementation, and other measures.

Handling these problems all at the same time is expensive and disruptive to your company. It's far better to anticipate issues that might result in a Form 483 and build your processes to avoid that scenario.

The most common causes of a 483 observation are:

Procedures not fully followed.

Poor investigations of discrepancies or failures (CAPA process not used).

Absence of written procedures.

Taking the time to be diligent with your written procedures can help prevent you from receiving a 483. **SOPs** (standard operating procedures) are required for **document control**, risk management, design controls, and many other aspects of device manufacturing.

Regulators want evidence that your company has outlined a way to handle these fundamental processes, otherwise they may issue a Form 483 observation. If you do receive a Form 483, there are a few rules around responding you should consider.

How To Respond To An FDA Form 483 Observation

Once you've received a Form 483 observation, you should ask to review the document with the FDA inspector. This will give you a better understanding of their concerns. You can streamline the inspection process by asking questions, coming to terms with the observations made, and identifying any potential errors in their observations.

You are obligated to respond to an FDA 483 observation in writing within 15 days. Before an inspector leaves your facility, you'll receive a draft of their inspection report (known as an Establishment Inspection Report, or EIR) as well as drafts of any 483 observations. They'll ask you whether you plan to address those observations, too.

Failure to demonstrate that the observed problems have been handled can result in an FDA warning letter. In our experience, companies who choose not to take action to resolve issues raised in a Form 483 observation tend to end up with a warning letter later on.

Remember, the FDA isn't messing around; if you receive a 483 observation, consider it to be fair warning that something isn't quite right with your internal processes and it may be worth your time to look into those issues further.

What Is An FDA Warning Letter?

An FDA warning letter is a formal notification from the FDA that identifies serious regulatory violations. A warning letter is issued by more senior FDA officials after they've reviewed the inspector's report. A warning letter is considered an escalation from a 483 observation.

The most common causes for an FDA warning letters are:

Non-compliant written procedures.

Failure to follow written procedures.

Failure to prove that regulations have been followed with adequate documentation.

Warning letters are typically delivered in person to ensure that they're viewed and handled promptly. Like with an FDA 483 observation, an FDA warning letter requires a written response within 15 days maximum. If the cause for the FDA warning letter is severe, the FDA may escalate the deadline. You are obligated to rectify the violations described in an FDA warning letter.

Warning letters are made public. Anyone can find that the company has been issued a letter. We've even heard of competitors using a company's warning letter as a negative example of why a potential customer should choose their own company over the competing one.

Like 483 observations, warning letters can be very expensive to deal with. Receiving a warning letter can significantly delay your time to market and consume capital in the process.

What's The Difference Between FDA 483 Observations And Warning Letters?

Let's recap. An FDA 483 observation is a notice that highlights potential regulatory problems, while a warning letter is an escalation of this notice. You need to respond in writing within 15 days of receiving both a 483 and a warning letter.

You're not obligated to handle observations cited by inspectors in a Form 483. However, it is inadvisable not to. You're far more likely to receive a warning letter if you don't address the FDA's concerns in the 483 observation.

If you receive a warning letter, you're required by law to make any changes necessary to satisfy the FDA's concerns. A warning letter is far more serious than a 483 observation. Any violations must be dealt with before you can meet compliance and bring your medical device to market.

It's also possible to receive 483 observations and warning letters at the same time. Usually, potential violations will be ordered in priority as determined by the investigator. It can take some careful managing to ensure you are getting done what the FDA expects of you.

ISO 13485 Equivalent To 483 Observations And Warning Letters

ISO is a little bit different in that they assess the severity of the situation (termed as a "non-conformance") and assign a "major or minor" value to it.

Each registrar has a slightly different process, but the expectation is that you'll communicate your corrective action plan within a set period of time. This period of time varies depending on whether the finding was minor or major.

As you conduct and complete the minor actions, these will usually be verified by the ISO auditor at your next audit, generally sometime within the next year. Anything major will need to be verified much sooner, possibly by a second onsite audit, or with a remote audit.

Major findings from an ISO audit could put your ISO certification at risk, as could persistently ignoring those minor observations. It's worth noting that one of the possible definitions falling under "major non-conformance" is "repeated nonconformities from previous audits."

There are some terminology differences between ISO and the FDA, for example, the term "observation" (which the FDA uses in place of non-conformance). For ISO audits, in addition to a nonconformity, an observation may be raised.

An observation is an isolated or non-systemic finding detected during an audit that does not require action to bring the system or any clause into compliance. It may also highlight a potential nonconformity.

An observation may also be a positive comment that informs you of some of the strengths of your system; whereas an observation from the FDA will always be something you need to improve or fix!

The following is an examination of the most commonly cited conditions that led to the issuance of Form 483s to drug companies last year (as summarized by the FDA in the most recent 12-month inspection period on record) accompanied by practical tips for avoiding them. It's important to note that while FY 2020 provided a smaller sample size from which trends could conclusively be derived (since fewer inspections were conducted during the height of the COVID-19 pandemic), the first four issues listed below consistently top the list of Form 483s issued to pharma companies year over year.

1. Discrepancies and/or Failures in Investigations (21 CFR 211.192)

The 21 CFR 211.192 guideline requires all deviations from written procedures to be thoroughly investigated and calls for adequate documentation of the results of those investigations. If a pharma company is unable to identify root causes and document them sufficiently, the FDA regards their internal investigations as incomplete. Failure to attentively investigate quality events can have catastrophic consequences for a pharma company's consumers, to say nothing of the long-term effects on product consistency, company reputation, and brand trust.

How to Avoid Observational Warnings for Investigational Failures:

Companies can dramatically simplify the investigation and documentation of quality events by implementing quality management system (QMS) software that automates the workflow of the entire corrective action/preventive action (CAPA) process — from initiation to investigation and all the way through to closure. Modern QMS solutions integrate CAPA-related data and documentation with other quality processes, which decreases the likelihood that information needed for investigations will slip through the cracks. Audit-ready written records of investigations can also be securely maintained within such a system, per compliance requirements.

2. Procedures Not in Writing or Not Fully Followed (21 CFR 211.22(d))

For a pharmaceutical company to provide evidence of compliance and commitment to safety, its standard operating procedures (SOPs) must be clearly written and maintained and modified in a timely and consistent manner. SOP records must be centrally located and readily available to investigators. When employees aren't given accurate or current written instructions for their tasks, or if they do not explicitly follow written instructions, mistakes and quality problems inevitably occur.

It's easy for companies to slip into such predicaments when disparate, paper-based document control systems are in use, or if the systems aren't capable of adequately tracking approvals, signatures, and audit trails. Up-to-date SOPs are more likely to go unnoticed if they're trapped in disconnected, siloed systems, which leads to a greater likelihood of employees executing their tasks using outdated work instructions.

How to Avoid SOP-Related Observational Warnings:

A proven digitized system can automate the routing and delivery of SOPs, policies, work instructions, and other pertinent documentation to designated personnel while maintaining SOPs and other critical documentation in a secure, web-based repository.

With digital systems, it's easy to see who has changed a document and when updates were made, which helps ensure that only the most current versions of SOPs are in use. Digitization also simplifies the search for and retrieval of audit-ready documentation.

3. Unsound Laboratory Controls (21 CFR 211.160(b))

Pharma companies must ensure that the specifications, standards, sampling plans, and test procedures for assuring that drug products conform to standards of identity, strength, quality, and purity are scientifically sound and appropriate.

While laboratory control infractions are often caused by what may initially seem to be only minor issues (e.g., inter-departmental communication miscues, disconnected processes, etc.), they can have disastrous ripple effects on product consistency and reputation.

Maintaining the integrity of laboratory controls requires the use of systems that effectively integrate multiple interrelated quality processes, particularly those critical to change control, nonconformance, document control, training, and CAPA.

How to Avoid Observational Warnings for Laboratory Control Failures:

An automated system that integrates related quality processes provides the most reliable means of maintaining sound laboratory controls. QMS software can connect every essential laboratory quality assurance process and prevent minor issues from snowballing into compliance failures. With digital, purpose-built solutions, companies gain the ability to automatically track documentation through collaboration, review, and approval steps and use it to apply timely controls where appropriate.

4. Absence of Written Procedures in Support of Production/Process Controls (21 CFR 211.100(a))

When deviations or other similar events are not adequately documented or tracked in pharma manufacturing environments, it's impossible to pinpoint root causes and take the appropriate corrective and/or preventive actions.

Many companies struggle to manage and control written procedures because the processes involved can be time consuming and cumbersome, especially if the organization is reliant on paper-based processes or if the documentation is scattered between multiple systems in different locales.

How Avoid Observational Warnings for Written Procedure Failures:

Pharma manufacturers can alleviate documentation inefficiencies by implementing a proven document management system with a track record of facilitating adherence to current good manufacturing practices (CGMP).

A digital, connected system streamlines documentation management and simplifies how it is controlled. Purpose-built software provides automated revision control and ensures that old versions of documents are archived in an inspection-ready state.

Any changes to production and process documentation can be initiated, escalated, and approved electronically, which provides greater assurance that critical documents are always going to the right person.

5. Lack of Appropriate Controls Over Computer Systems (21 CFR 211.68(b))

The FDA reported 57 instances of computer system control deficiencies in FY 2020, marking the first time the issue has cracked the list of the top five most observed Form 483 infractions.

This surge isn't surprising, given the FDA's increasing focus on data integrity and data management matters in general.

It stands to reason that these types of data-related issues will only continue to get more attention from inspectors in the future, and trends indicate that data managed electronically via laboratory instrumentation and manufacturing batch records poses a particular ongoing concern to the agency.

How to Avoid Observational Warnings for Inadequate Computer System Controls:

Since Section 211.68(b) mandates that only authorized personnel may institute changes to master production, control, and other records, pharma companies must have reliable systems in place that prohibit interference by unauthorized users.

Organizations that rely on paper-based systems never have the assurance that only authorized users have altered records. With a proven electronic batch record (EBR) software system, access to records can be restricted as needed. Plus, if the software is cloud-based, authorized users have anytime/anywhere access to records, which maximizes efficiency.

To learn more about FDA expectations and how your organization can avoid the types of quality failures that lead to **Form 483s**, download the "Overcoming Pharma's Top 6 Quality and Compliance Oversights" industry brief.

Final Thoughts

If you've received an FDA 483 observation or an FDA warning letter, you need to handle the situation with care. The same is true for dealing with non-conformances from an ISO audit.

These noncompliant incidences can have serious implications for your company and its ability to save and improve lives with medical devices. Listening to what regulatory bodies require for the production of safe and effective devices is always the best practice.

One of the reasons we created Greenlight Guru's QMS software for medical devices is to help companies navigate these issues with ease. Our medical device nonconformance management software was designed to allow you to reduce non-conformance cycle times and manage issues that are identified within your quality system.

Our audit management software helps you conduct internal audits with ease, route findings to the right place based on risk, and easily share results. Both of these are useful aspects of our medical device QMS, created to improve the way you handle noncompliance at your company.

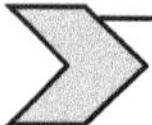

Conclusion

From the above stated study, it is concluded that the market complaints and the product recalls will decrease the reputation and brand image of the firm. They should be addressed in a proper way with the predetermined working procedures. All these things should be documented using specified format and should be compiled for the future references. The FDA-483 will help to record these complaints and recall procedures and their results. Also it will help in the assurance of import and the export.

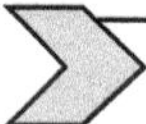

Important Questions

1. Why it is important for pharmaceutical companies to comply with the market complaints?

2. What is the difference between internal complaints and external complaints?

3. Classify the complaints according to its major components.

4. What happens when any pharmaceutical company gets Form 483?

5. What is Form 483? What are the next steps after getting Form 483?

6. What is the difference between FDA Form 483 and warning letter?

7. What are the different stages of handling the market complaints?

8. Briefly explain the investigation that is carried out while handling the market complaint.

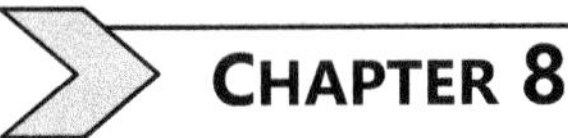

CHAPTER 8

Pharmaceutical Quality Audits

Audits are conducted to ascertain the validity and reliability of the information; also to provide an assessment of the internal control of a system. It provides management with information on the efficiency with which the company controls the quality of its processes and products.

The audit in simple terms could be defined as the inspection of a process or a system to ensure that it meets the requirements of its intended use. International organization for standardization (ISO) defines the audits as "Systematic, independent and documented process for obtaining audit evidence and evaluating them objectively to determine the degree to which the verification criteria are met.

Instead of considering the audit as an intrusive and potentially threatening review, pharmacies should consider the audit as a quality control mechanism. The results of the audit and the resulting corrective actions ensure all the involved parties that a program works in accordance with established rules of practice.

In the pharmaceutical industry, audits are virtual means for assessing compliance with the established objectives defined in the quality system and thus paving the way for the continuous improvement program by providing feedback to management. A company that produces drugs today must be able to demonstrate that it does so with absolute reliability, in optimal conditions and with extreme uniformity that allows accurate reproduction . In food and drug administration (FDA) and ISO environments, auditing of both compliance and performance is essential.

Pharmaceutical audit experience includes the drafting and revision of validation policies, guidelines and standard operating procedures (SOP) from project qualification to performance evaluation phases. If implemented correctly; it can be one of the most effective means of improvement.

Definition of internal audit

The chartered institute of management accountants, UK (CIMA) defines Internal Audit as: 'An independent appraisal activity established within an organization as a service to it. It is a control which functions by examining and evaluating the adequacy and effectiveness of other controls; a management tool which analyses the effectiveness of all parts of an organization's operations and management.' The Institute of Internal Auditors (IIA) also defines Internal Audit on similar lines as: 'Internal auditing is an independent, objective assurance and consulting activity designed to add value and improve an organization's operations.

It helps an organization accomplish its objectives by bringing a systematic, disciplined approach to evaluate and improve the effectiveness of risk management, control, and governance processes.' These definitions state two clear functions of the Internal Audit activity namely; Internal control: A process which is performed by the employees of the company as well as the information technology systems that are used to assist the company in achieving its objectives.

Management tool

These monitors and evaluates the effectiveness of operational processes and risk management of a company.

Goals of an audit

The simple goal of this complex process is to evaluate existing activities and documentation and determine if they meet the established standards. An audit will evaluate the strengths and weaknesses of quality control and quality assurance processes, the results of which will help us to improve processes and build a better system for the benefit of the company.

Every product manufactured by a pharmaceutical company has characteristics that must be quantified or qualified by laboratory tests. Quality control and quality assurance are the necessary processes that play the role of control and balance system in pharmaceutical industry.

With proper preparation and planning, the audit itself must easily achieve the intended purpose. Effective auditing and proper compliance with standards will help build brand reputation and avoid the negative effects of non-compliance, such as fines, bad public relations and court proceedings.

Objectives

Audit objectives may include,

- Evaluating conformity of requirements to ISO 9001
- Evaluating conformity of documentation to ISO 9001
- Judging conformity of implementation to documentation
- Determining effectiveness in meeting requirements and objectives
- Meeting any contractual or regulatory requirements for auditing
- Providing an opportunity to improve the quality management system

- Permitting registration and inclusion in a list of registered companies

- Qualifying potential suppliers

Audits and regulatory standards

The ISO, a global leader in the development of international standards, is instrumental in boosting interest in quality audits among manufacturers and other types of businesses when it published the ISO 9000 standards in 1987.

Today, popular standards such as ISO 9001: 2000, ISO 14001:2004, and ISO 13485 all require internal audits of the quality system (or the environmental management system in the case of ISO 14001: 2004).

Under these standards, audit serves as a mechanism for evaluating and improving quality. The same principle is reflected in a number of regulations enforced by the Food and Drug Administration. Under the Quality System Regulation (21 Code of federal regulations [CFR] Part 820), medical device manufacturers are required to conduct audits to ensure that the quality system is compliant (Sec. 820.22).

The current good manufacturing practice (CGMP) regulations for pharmaceuticals (21 CFR Parts 210-211) and for blood and blood components (21 CFR Part 606) include general requirements for regular evaluation of quality standards. Guidance for the pharmaceutical industry and blood establishments also emphasize the importance of audits. For example, the "Guidance for Industry Quality Systems Approach to Pharmaceutical CGMP Regulations" recommends internal audits and supplier audits.

The "Guidelines for Quality Assurance in Blood Establishments" call for a comprehensive audit of the quality assurance program . Benefits of auditing whilst there is usually low influence on regulatory inspections, audits should be seen as a management tool to assess the company's in-house quality management system. Internal, as well as external auditing, can help to achieve this goal. The major benefits of an effective audit system can be summarized as follows:

- Managing a quality management system

- Detecting in advance weak points, through identification of unsatisfactory trends or situations

- Preventing quality failures, on the basis of quality data reviewing

- Informing Senior Management about the quality level of facilities and/or operations

- Standardizing audits will optimize the output, the quality level of audits will increase (and therefore the quality of products and services) which will finally lead to a continuous improvement loop.

- The auditee will understand that audits are not created to control and criticize his work, but will improve the company's performance. This will lead to a higher acceptance of the audits. He will see audits as a chance to educate and improve his knowledge in terms of quality related aspects.

- Combining audits of quality, safety, and environmental matters will reduce the number of audits significantly which will give a greater acceptance to the auditee and will save his time.

- Additional benefits can be achieved by pooling audits, for example, Shared Third Party Audits.

- By establishing a high-quality audit system throughout the industry, the level of compliance will increase. Mutual confidence building and an improved relationship between the partners will be the result of these efforts.

Types of audits

The quality audit system mainly classified in three different categories

A. Internal Audits

B. External Audits

C. Regulatory Audits

Quality audits are performed to verify the effectiveness of a quality management system. This type of audit is also known as First-Party Audit or self-audit. Those auditing and those being audited all belong to the same organization.

A. Internal audits

Internal audit is a professional activity that consists of advising organizations on how to achieve their goals in a better way. The internal audit involves the use of a systematic methodology to analyze business processes or organizational problems and recommend solutions. The main objectives of internal audits can be summarized as follows:

1. To assist the internal control system.
2. Review of organizational policies and their operations.
3. Verify the accuracy and authenticity of errors and frauds.
4. Detection and prevention of errors and faults.
5. Safeguarding the assets
6. Applicability of accounting policies.
7. Helps in smooth functioning of the internal check system.
8. In a pharmaceutical facility for internal auditing, one requires to check mainly two things namely, Activities carried out by different departments and Documents maintained by these departments. For this

purpose, a department-wise questionnaire and document list is required to be prepared in detail. This type of audit is also known as Second-Party Audit. It refers to a customer conducting an audit on a supplier or contractor. Although there are no strict legal requirements for this control. It is always advisable to evaluate the competence of the contractors in which we produce our products or carry out the analysis of our products or any other activity according to GMP.

9. Performing these audits also offers important commercial advantages:

B. External audits

1. Develop knowledge and confidence in the partnership agreement

2. Ensures that requirements are understood and met

3. Allow the reduction of some activities (e. g. in-house quality control (QC) testing of starting materials)

4. Reduce the risk of failure (and, by implication, its costs)

C. Regulatory Audits

Many pharmaceutical industry suppliers are ISO 9001 or ISO 9002-certified and are regularly audited by their certification body. Pharmaceutical contract manufacturing or packaging companies will need to be licensed and will be subject to regulatory audits.

This type of audit is also known as Third-Party Audit. Neither customer nor supplier conducts this type of audit. A regulatory agency or independent body conducts a third party audit for compliance or certification or registration purposes. International regulatory bodies such as. Medicines and healthcare products regulatory agency (MHRA), UK, United States food and drug administration (USFDA), Therapeutic goods administration (TGA), Australia, South Africa Health Product Regulatory Agency (SAHPRA), Medicines control council (MCC), South Africa, etc. are responsible for carrying out these checks. There is a team of Regulatory to perform the audit; it must be composed of audit inspectors and a multidisciplinary company team.

The company must have representatives from each of the following departments: production, quality control, warehouse, maintenance, administration/personnel and marketing/sales.

These audits can be performed without warning (MHRA currently performs around ten percent of its inspections in the UK in this way) as manufacturers are required to always comply with GMPs.

Regulatory bodies in other countries where products are sold can also audit companies (e. g. FDA audits European manufacturers). All regulatory inspectors are extensively trained, competent and professional. All MHRA inspectors are professionally qualified and have a minimum of five years of appropriate experience in a production operation; they will be in the registers of persons eligible to act as qualified persons and lead auditors. Failure to approve a regulatory audit may result in restrictions (or revocation) of production or import/export license. (The FDA has recently imposed "punitive consensus decrees" on financial companies that did not respond adequately to the audit results and comply with the GMPs).

Therefore, it is essential that companies have defined processes for managing audits and staff should be adequately trained for being audited. Internal audits can provide valuable opportunities for practice .

Principles of auditing

The audit is characterized by dependence on a number of principles. These principles should help to establish audit as an effective and reliable tool to support management policies and controls, by providing information on what an organization can act to improve its performance.

Adherence to these principles is a prerequisite in order to provide relevant and sufficient audit conclusions and allow auditors to work independently from each other, to reach similar conclusions in similar circumstances.

Integrity

The basis of professionalism: The auditors and the person who administers an audit program must:

Carry out their work with honesty, diligence, and responsibility;

Observe and comply with applicable legal requirements;

Demonstrate their competence while carrying out their work;

Be sensitive to any influence that can be exercised on the judgment while conducting an audit.

Fair presentation

The obligation to report truthfully and accurately : The audit findings, audit conclusions and audit reports should truthfully and accurately reflect the activities of the audit. Significant obstacles encountered during the audit and unresolved diverging opinions between the audit team and the auditee should be reported. The communication should be truthful, accurate, objective, timely, clear and complete.

Due professional care: the application of diligence and judgment in auditing Auditors should pay due attention to the importance of the task they perform and the trust placed in them by the audit client and other interested parties. An important factor in the execution of work with due professional attention is having the ability to express reasoned judgments in all audit situations.

Confidentiality: security of information Auditors should exercise discretion in the use and protection of information acquired in the course of exercising their duties. Audit information should not be used inappropriately for personal gain by the auditor or the audit client, or in a manner detrimental to the legitimate interests of the auditee. This concept includes the correct management of sensitive or confidential information.

Independence: The basis for the impartiality of the audit and the objectivity of the audit conclusions The auditors should be independent of the activity audited wherever possible, and in all cases, they should act in a manner that is free from prejudice and conflicts of interest.

For internal audits, auditors must be independent of the operational managers of the function being audited. Auditors must maintain objectivity throughout the review process to ensure that audit findings and conclusions are based only on audit evidence. For small organizations, internal auditors may not be totally independent of the activity being audited, but all efforts must be made to eliminate bias and encourage objectivity.

Evidence-based approach: the rational method for achieving reliable and reproducible audit conclusions in a systematic audit process Audit evidence must be verifiable. In general, it will be based on samples of available information, since an audit is conducted in a limited period of time and with limited resources. An appropriate use of sampling should be applied, as it is closely related to the confidence that can be included in the audit conclusions .

The auditor within the audit system : An auditor is defined by ISO 19011 as a person with the competence to perform an audit. To perform an audit, the auditor must be authorized for that particular audit. Auditor's responsibility

The auditor has the following responsibilities:

- Assist in the selection of the team and inform the team
- Responsibility to plan and manage all phases of the audit
- Represent the audit team with the auditee
- Control conflicts and manage difficult situations
- Direct and control all meetings with the team and the auditee
- Make decisions about audit issues and the quality system
- Report the results of the audit without delay
- Report the main obstacles encountered
- Report critical non-conformances immediately
- Possesses effective communication skills

Managing an audit program: An audit program may include one or more audits, depending on the size, nature, and complexity of the organization to be audited. These audits may have a variety of objectives and may also include joint (multiple auditing organizations) or combined (Quality management and Environmental management systems) audits.

Management of an audit program includes all the activities necessary for planning and organizing the types and number of audits, and for providing resources for conducting them effectively and efficiently within the specified time frames.

The organization's top management should grant the authority for managing the audit program. Those assigned the responsibility for managing the audit program should:

1. Plan, establish, implement, monitor, review and improve the audit program
2. Identify the necessary resources and ensure they are provided. Managing an audit program–process flow.

The planning and conducting of audit activities involve the following process flow or life cycle.

What is information?

Information is simply the facts or knowledge provided or learned. It can be tacit, in people's heads, or explicit, in documents-electronic or hard copy . During the audit, information relevant to the objectives, scope and criteria, including information on interfaces between functions, activities and processes, should be collected by appropriate sampling and should be verified.

Only verifiable information can be audit evidence which must be recorded. Audit evidence is any information used by the auditor to determine if the audited information is in accordance with the established criteria and to arrive at the conclusions on which the audit opinion is based.

Internal Audit

Evidence includes any data, information, process flows, vouchers, bills, memos, contracts or transactions. The internal audit evidence collected would be dependent on the following:

Audit procedures to use-specific procedures should be spelled out for instruction during the audit.

Sample size-how many items should be tested for each audit procedure.

Items to select-determine which items in the population should be selected.

Timing-timing can vary from the beginning of the accounting period to the closure of it. Methods of gathering audit information. There are six basic methods of gathering information during an audit. Depending on the type of information that needs to be obtained, the Internal Auditor will need to determine which method, or combination of methods, should be used.

Interviews

Interviewing is a powerful data collection technique, which works well on its own and is often used to support other techniques, such as observation. The interviewee's insights can guide the Internal Auditor's decisions about what to observe. The most important thing to remember when interviewing is to always talk to the right person, as it can save a lot of time and confusion. Communication is a key element to the success of any audit. The more effectively the Internal Auditor interviews personnel, the more useful information will be gathered.

Questions may be asked several times in different ways or to different people depending on their level of responsibility (Operator, Supervisor, etc.) in order to get a complete answer.

Inspections

When inspecting something, it is good practice to start with general observations and then proceeding to the more specific elements. First, the Internal Auditor will have a good overall look around the facility and then examine specific items more closely, noting anything that does not seem quite right. It is important to ask questions throughout the inspection. If a problem is found, the Internal Auditor must investigate (dig deeper) to explore the extent of the finding.

Reviewing documents

When reviewing company records, the Internal Auditor can use a number of techniques. Random sampling is one of them. It gives a general idea of the quality of record keeping and exposes the potential problem areas. However, one sample taken in one given period of time is usually not enough to form accurate conclusions. Another important aspect of record keeping is clarity.

Documents should be clear regardless of who reads them. Details vary but, in general, every document should carry a title, an owner and a revision status. If any of this information is missing, the Internal Auditor should ask why.

The revisions noted should be checked against the master record. Changes must be authorized, signed and dated by an authorized person.

Observations

The simplest way to check how a process works is to observe it in action. Observing a routine activity for a couple of hours can give the Internal Auditor the opportunity to see how something is done under normal circumstances.

He or she should ask questions about what they see, making sure at all times not to interfere with the processes they are observing, as that may cause the personnel not to carry out their tasks as they usually do.

Vertical tracking

This method is also referred to as "vertical auditing" and consists of following a specific development from the beginning until the end, simultaneously checking all the records that are produced in the process.

Applying the vertical tracking technique can lead the Internal Auditor to areas that were not initially part of the scope, but it does facilitate a bigger picture view, as this allows the Internal Auditor to see how the various parts of a given program work together.

Exercises

The aim of an exercise is to test something that is usually done at the facility as part of the routine. However, the Internal Auditor gets to pick the time and the circumstances for the test. The subject of testing can be the personnel, the program, or the equipment.

An Internal Auditor should not run an exercise without the knowledge and cooperation of the auditee. Doing so is likely to have negative consequences as unannounced actions may breach certain facility specific rules or regulations which the Internal Auditor is unaware of.

Taking notes

A good Internal Auditor must have his or her own efficient way of taking notes. This is an extremely important part of the job that cannot be neglected. Notes must get reviewed and refined along the way. In situations where taking notes is inconvenient, a mental notetaking technique should be used. Notes are used to organize thoughts and observations which will, in turn, help the Internal Auditor reach accurate conclusions throughout the audit.

Notes need to be reviewed and completed at the end of each audit day. process for collecting information to reach audit conclusions.

Administration

The internal audit team must have the confidence and trust of the key stakeholders it works with and be seen as a credible source of assurance and advice. This confidence should not be assumed and can only be established and maintained by having an effective working relationship, by delivering high-quality and timely advice and internal audit reports that are seen to be contributing directly to assisting the organization to meet its responsibilities. The key stakeholders of internal audit are:

- Chief Executive
- Board of Directors
- Audit Committee

- Senior management
- External auditor

Other reviewers

The importance of these individual relationships is analysed below.

Chief executive

While internal audit reports functionally to the Audit Committee, it is important that the Head of Internal Audit has direct access, as and when required, to the Chief Executive.

Organisations today, recognize the advantages in making the Head of Internal Audit directly accountable to the Chief Executive. This not only sends a clear signal about the importance of the internal audit function, it also facilitates regular contact between the Chief Executive and internal audit. This contact should be used as an opportunity to gain insights into new and emerging risks and issues facing the organisation and to discuss the role the Chief Executive expects internal audit to fulfill in the company.

Board of directors

The Head of Internal Audit may formally report to the Board of Directors on the effectiveness of the internal audit function in order to exchange views and ideas. As the Audit Committee is usually a sub-committee of the Board, this responsibility is often delegated to the Audit Committee. As a minimum, it is important that the Head of Internal Audit has direct access to the Chair of the Board and the Chief Executive, as and when required.

Audit committee

Audit Committees play an integral role in the governance framework of organizations. It assists Chief Executives and Boards to understand whether key controls are appropriate and operating effectively.

In this respect, the relationship between internal audit and the Audit Committee is crucial and has a number of dimensions which are mentioned below:

(a) Advise the Chief Executive about the internal audit plans of the organisation;

(b) Direct or coordinate work programs relating to internal and external audits;

(c) Review the content of internal [and external] audits to identify significant matters of concern, and to advise the Chief Executive on good practice or opportunities for improvement;

(d) Review the adequacy of responses to reports of internal and external audits;

(e) Endorse the internal audit charter and be responsible for either reviewing and approving internal audit plans or recommending their approval by the Chief Executive/Board of Directors;

(f) Act as the internal audit function's primary client and form a sound professional relationship with the internal audit team as a whole and each of its members;

(g) Utilize internal audit reports and its general interaction with the Internal Audit team, to assess the effectiveness of controls and the performance of the organisation and

(h) Utilize the internal audit function to undertake secretariat compliance given this relationship, it is important that both formal and informal lines of communication be maintained between internal audit and the Audit Committee and with individual committee members, particularly the Chair. Audit Committee members should be in a position to be able to openly discuss matters of interest with the Head of Internal Audit.

It is also good practice for the Audit Committee to meet privately with the Head of Internal Audit from time to time to ask questions and to seek feedback from internal audit without management being present. This practice also supports the independent role of internal audit.

Senior management

To effectively fulfill its responsibilities, it is important that internal audit has a professional and constructive relationship with senior management of the organization.

Internal auditors should interact on a regular basis with members of the senior management team, and through the delivery of practical, business-focused and useful reports and advice, build a relationship that is based on cooperation, collaboration and mutual respect. Meetings with organization managers should be used as an opportunity to be briefed on key business developments and associated risks facing the organization. These meetings should also be used to obtain informal feedback about the performance of internal audit and to assist in identifying ways that internal audit can best assist organization management.

Thus, the internal audit team would encourage managers to seek their advice and assistance on either an informal or formal basis as the need arises.

External auditors

External auditors too must help in developing internal audit strategy and internal audit work plan. Both audit teams need to address the key financial and business systems underpinning the company's financial statements and to avoid duplication of compliance and assurance. To avoid such duplication, the external auditor must evaluate the work of the internal audit function to determine its adequacy for external audit purposes. The Internal audit function can be made responsible for liaising with external auditor on behalf of the organization. Such a role can be a useful way for an internal audit team to be aware of planned and actual external audit coverage.

Thus, a constructive relationship between both sets of auditors assists in the conduct of external audits. Such a role can only be fulfilled when there is healthy communication between internal and external audit teams which can be achieved by setting up formally establish meetings between internal and external audit to allow for a routine exchange of information.

Other reviewers

Internal audit is one of a number of internal and external review and assurance activities that exist as part of an organization's governance arrangements. The company shall benefit when all these activities, such as those performed by the Ombudsman and regulators, operate in a coordinated and complementary manner to the greatest extent possible. This requires regular formal and informal contact between review bodies to minimize duplication and overlap.

Some organisations see a benefit in protocols being formalised for such activities: providing, for example, for the regular exchange of views and information and for the reporting of the results of work undertaken in a coordinated manner. Protocols can be particularly important in situations where internal audit needs to work closely with other entities as a result of inter-agency or other agreements.

Audit planning procedures

In order to conduct an audit effectively and efficiently, the work needs to be planned and controlled. The form and nature of the planning required for an audit will be affected by the size and complexity of the enterprise, the commercial environment in which it operates, the methods of processing transactions and the reporting requirements to which it is subjected.

Audit planning is the formulation of the general strategy for audit which sets the direction for the audit, describes the expected scope and conduct of the audit and provides guidance for the development of the audit program.

Adequate planning of an audit work aims at

(a) Establishing the intended means of achieving the objectives of the audit

(b) Assisting in the direction and control of the work

(c) Helping to ensure that attention is devoted to critical aspects of the audit work

(d)   Ensuring that the work is completed expeditiously

(e)   Facilitating review of the audit work

(f)   Helping to assign the proper tasks to members of the audit team and coordinates outside experts.

The audit plan

The auditor should develop an audit plan for the audit in order to reduce audit risk to an acceptably low level. The audit plan is more detailed than the overall audit strategy and includes the nature, timing, and extent of audit procedures to be performed by engagement team members in order to obtain sufficient appropriate audit evidence to reduce audit risk to an acceptably low level. Documentation of the audit plan also serves as a record of the proper planning and performance of the audit procedures that can be reviewed and approved prior to the performance of further audit procedures.

Planning objectives

"The objective of the auditor is to plan the audit so that it will be performed in an effective manner." Audits are potentially complex, risky and expensive processes. Although firms have internal manuals and standardized procedures, it is vital that engagements are planned to ensure that the auditor:

- Devotes appropriate attention to important areas of the audit;

- Identifies and resolves potential problems on a timely basis

- Organizes and manages the audit so that it is performed in an effective and efficient manner;

- Selects team members with appropriate capabilities and competencies;

- Directs and supervises the team and reviews their work; and

- Effectively coordinates the work of others, such as experts and internal audit. The purpose of all this is to ensure that the risk of performing a poor quality audit (and ultimately giving an inappropriate audit opinion) is reduced to an acceptable level

The steps in planning an audit include

Planning Procedures : Basic discussions with the client

About the nature of the engagement are performed first, and the auditor meets the key employees or new employees of a continuing client. The overall audit strategy or the timing of the audit may also be discussed.

Review of audit documentation from previous audits performed by the accounting firm or a predecessor auditor (if the latter makes these audit documentation available) will assist in developing an outline of the audit program.

Ask about recent developments .in the company such as mergers and new product lines which will cause the audit to differ from earlier years. Interim financial statements are analyzed to identify accounts and transactions that differ from expectations (based on factors such as budgets or prior periods). The performance of such analytical procedures is mandatory

In the planning of an audit to identify accounts that may be misstated and that deserve special emphasis in the audit program. Non-audit personnel

Of the accounting firm who have provided services (such as tax preparation) to the client should be identified and consulted to learn more about the client.

Staffing : for the audit should be determined and a meeting held to discuss the engagement.

Timing : of the various audit procedures should be determined Outside assistance needs should be determined, including the use of a specialist The internal audit work plan would generally include: is needed to coordinate activities.

1. Audit title
2. Functional and Operational Area to be covered
3. Director and manager responsible
4. Type and scope of internal audit
5. The benefit expected by the audit procedure
6. Resources allocation for the purpose of the audit
7. Proposed duration and timelines for completion

Auditing procedure

There are total 10 steps of the audit process:

Notification

Audit process begins with notification. The notification process alerts the party to be audited of the date and time of the process. The notification also will list the documents that the order wishes to review in order to understand the organization of the company.

Planning

Planning is the steps the auditor takes, before the audit, to identify key areas of risk and areas of concern.

Opening meeting

Meeting between the auditing staff and senior management of the auditing target as well as administrative staff. The auditors will describe the process they will undertake. Management will describe areas of concern to them and the schedule of the employees that must be consulted.

Fieldwork

Fieldwork begins after the results of the meeting are used to adjust the final audit plans. Employees are notified of the audit, schedules are drawn up regarding the activities of the audit staff, and an initial investigation begun after learning of business procedures, interviewing key staff, testing current business practices by sampling, reviewing the law and testing internal rules and practices for reasonableness.

Communication

The audit team should consistently be in contact with the corporate auditor to clarify processes, gain access to documents and clarify procedures.

Draft audit

At the completion of the audit, the next step, the draft audit, is prepared. The draft audit detail what was done and what was found, a distribution list of parties to receive preliminary results, and a list of concerns.

Management response

The draft is given to management to review, edit and suggest changes, probe areas of concern and correct errors. Upon making final corrections, the report is given to management for the seventh step, the management response. Management is requested to answer the report by stating whether they agree with the problems cited, the plan to correct noted problem and the expected date by which all issues will have been addressed.

Final meeting

The final meeting is designed to close loose ends, discuss the management response and address the scope of the audit.

Report distribution

The ninth step is the report distribution, where the final audit report is sent to appropriate officials inside and outside the audit area.

Feedback

The last step is the audit feedback whereby the audited company implements the recommended changes and the auditor's review and test the quality, adherence and effects of the adopted changes. This continues until all issues are adopted and the next audit cycle begins.

As the audit proceeds, there might arise some situations where the facts indicate there is a failure, either partially or wholly, of the quality management system, such a situation is called Recording nonconformities or deficiencies nonconformity". a condition adverse to Quality

What is nonconformity?

The non-fulfillment of a requirement

1. The procedure or defined process does not conform to the regulatory requirements. There may be nonconformity for one of three reasons

2. The procedure or process has not been put into practice in the described way

3. The practice, what is actually done, is not effective (planned results not achieved). The statement of nonconformity needs to be in a format understandable both to people in the audit and to those who were not. People who were not present at the audit will be assigned to take the necessary corrective action most often. This need alone defines some rules for the recording of nonconformities:

    1. Exact observation of the facts. Only the facts are needed, and the reporting of them needs to be exact.

    2. Where was it found? The statement needs to identify exactly where it was found; otherwise, it may not be found again.

    3. What was found? It needs to be clear so that people understand what aspect of the system is nonconforming.

    4. Why is it nonconformity? The statement needs to make it clear what specified requirement has not been met.

    5. What is the objective evidence of the nonconformity? What audit evidence do we have–records, documents, statements or observations for our nonconformity findings?

    6. Who was involved? The statement often has no need to involve specific people, but where the objective evidence was based on a statement, and then the statement and the originator (s) need to be clear. Job titles rather than names should be used.

    7. Use local terminology.

    8. Industry has its own names for certain activities, documents, etc. These unique terms should be used for clarity.

    9. Make it retrievable. Someone has to go back after the audit and put it right, possibly after a considerable period of time.

    10. Make it helpful. To be helpful, nonconformity statements should be complete, correct, concise and clear. Suggestions, particularly on external audits, are not recommended, nor are they the auditor's duty

Classification of deficiencies

The number of nonconformities that can arise during an audit can be numerous. Following types of defects are identified during an internal audit and these are helpful in regulatory compliance: Critical defect

Critical defects have a high probability of resulting in a product recall or in an adverse physiological response by the consumer. Critical deficiencies found in internal audits that usually produce significant effects on the strength, identity, safety, and purity of the product that will be considered during regulatory compliance.

The possible source of a critical defect

- Cross-contamination of materials of the product
- Incorrect labeling
- Active ingredients outside of specifications
- Product manufactured according to obsolete or unapproved procedures
- Open sterile products located in a non-aseptic area
- Untrained operators working in the sterile filling area
- Contaminated purified water or water for injection system Major defect Major defects found during the internal audit can reduce the usability or stability of a product, but without causing harm to the consumer. The possible source of a major defect
- Major equipment not calibrated or out of calibration
- Inadequate segregation of quarantine components
- Inadequate evaluation of production process outside of action levels
- Process deviations not properly documented or investigated
- Operator not trained in or familiar with the standard operating procedures
- Preventive maintenance on a critical water system not conducted according to schedule
- Lack of standard operating procedures for cleaning equipment.
- Audits of a contract manufacturer not conducted Minor defect Minor defects have a low probability of affecting the quality or usability of the product which can help in regulatory compliance. Possible source of the minor defect
- Failure to complete all batch record entries
- Warehouse not cleaned according to schedule
- Cracks in wall surfaces
- Failures to correct documentation errors properly
- Operator uniform not properly worn
- Standard operating procedure review is overdue
- Adhesive tape used on manufacturing equipment
- Laboratory buffer solutions are obsolete

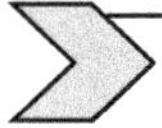 ## Conclusion

A quality systems approach calls for audits to be conducted at planned intervals to evaluate effective implementation and maintenance of the quality system and to determine if processes and products meet established parameters and specifications. An audit performed by a well-trained and thoroughly prepared auditor can be highly beneficial by identifying areas for genuine improvement.

An audit should not to be seen as interrogation with the auditee as permanent loser, it is a comparison of what is laid down to what is in place. Auditing is no goal in itself. Auditing in the pharmaceutical sector serves two different categories: regulatory compliance and business needs.

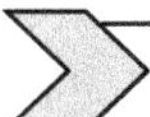 ## Important Questions

1. Why Quality audits form an important part of pharmaceutical company?

2. Highlight the goals with which quality audits are carried out.

3. Whose job is it to carry out the audit trial review in the laboratory?

4. What are the objectives of the pharma quality audits?

5. Who is responsible to carry out internal audits in the pharmaceutical organization?

6. What is the difference between Internal Audit and External Audit? Explain.

7. What are the principles of Audit? Explain with example.

8. Who is an auditor? Highlight his role and responsibilities towards carrying out audits.

CHAPTER 9

USFDA Guidelines-Process Validation

Validation is the most recognized and important parameter of GMPs. This article provide introduction about the process validation of pharmaceutical manufacturing process and its importance according to The U.S. Food and Drug Administration (FDA). This work is to present an introduction and general overview on process validation of pharmaceutical manufacturing process. Quality cannot be ensured by sampling, testing, release of materials and products. Quality assurance techniques must be used to build the quality into the product at every step and not just tested for at the end. Process validation of a process will ensure production of drug of reproducible quality. In pharmaceutical industry, Process Validation performs this task to build the quality into the product because according to ISO 9000:2000, it had proven to be an important tool for quality management of pharmaceuticals.

The concept of validation was first proposed by two Food and Drug Administration (FDA) officials, Ted Byers and Bud Loftus, in the mid 1970's in order to improve the quality of pharmaceuticals. The first validation activities were focused on the processes involved in making these products, but quickly spread to associated processes including environmental control, media fill, equipment sanitization and purified water production.

In a guideline, validation is act of demonstrating and documenting that any procedure, process, and activity will consistently lead to the expected results. It includes the qualification of systems and equipment. The goal of the validation is to ensure that quality is built into the system at every step, and not just tested for at the end, as such validation activities will commonly include training on production material and operating procedures, training of people involved and monitoring of the system whilst in production. In general, an entire process is validated and a particular object within that process is verified. The regulations also set out an expectation that the different parts of the production process are well defined and controlled, such that the results of that production will not substantially change over time.

Why to Validate a process?

The main reasons for validation are

1. **Quality assurance:** Quality cannot be assured by daily quality control testing because of the limitations of statistical samples and the limited

facilities of finished product testing. Validation checks the accuracy and reliability of a system or a process to meet the predetermined criteria. A successful validation provides high degree of assurance that a consistent level of quality is maintained in each unit of the finished product from one batch to another batch.

2. **Economics:** Due to successful validation, there is a decrease in the sampling and testing procedures and there are less number of product rejections and retesting. This lead to cost- saving benefits.

3. **Compliance:** For compliance to current good manufacturing practices CGMPs, validation is essential.

Department Responsible:

1. **Site validation committee (SVC):** Develop Site master Validation plan, Prepare/execute/approve validation Studies

2. **Manufacturing department:** Prepares the batches as a routine Production batch

3. **Quality assurance:** Ensure compliance, see that documentations/ procedures are in place, approves protocols and reports

4. **Quality control:** Perform testing and reviews protocol and report as needed.

Responsible Authorities for Validation: The validation working party is convened to define progress, coordinate and ultimately, approve the entire effort, including all of the documentation generated. The working party would usually include the following staff members, preferably those with a good insight into the company's operation.

1. Head of quality assurance

2. Head of engineering

3. Validation manager

4. Production manager

5. Specialist validation discipline: all areas

Elements of Validation:

Qualification is pre-requisite of validation. The qualification includes the following:

1. **Design Qualification (DQ):** In this qualification, compliance of design with GMP should be demonstrated. The principles of design should be such as to achieve the objectives of GMP with regard to equipment. Mechanical drawings and design features provided by the manufacturer of the equipment should be examined.

2. **Installation Qualification (IQ):** Installation qualification should be carried out on new or modified facilities, systems and equipment. The following main points should be includes in the installation qualification.

   Checking of installation of equipment, piping, services and instrumentation.

   Collection of supplier's operating working instructions and maintenance requirements and their calibration requirements.

   Verification of materials of construction

   Sources of spares and maintenance

3. **Operational Qualification (OQ):** Operational qualification should follow IQ, OQ should include the following:

   Tests developed from the knowledge of the processes systems and equipment.

   Defining lower and upper operating limits. Sometimes, these are called 'worst case' conditions.

4. **Performance Qualification (PQ):** After IQ and OQ have been completed, the next qualification that should be completed is PQ. PQ should include the following:

   Tests using production materials, substitutes or simulated product. These can be developed from the knowledge of the process and facilities, systems or equipment.

   Tests to include conditions with upper and lower limits

Process Validation

The U.S. Food and Drug Administration (FDA) has proposed guidelines with the following definition for process validation: Process validation is establishing documented evidence which provides a high degree of assurance that a specific process (such as the manufacture of pharmaceutical dosage forms) will consistently produce a product meeting its predetermined specifications and quality characteristics. According to the FDA, assurance of product quality is derived from careful and systemic attention to a number of important factors, including: selection of quality components and materials, adequate product and process design, and (statistical) control of the process through in-process and end-product testing. Thus, it is through careful design (qualification) and validation of both the process and its control systems that a high degree of confidence can be established that all individual manufactured units of a given batch or succession of batches that meet specifications will be acceptable.

This guidance describes process validation activities in three stages.

Stage 1 – Process Design: The commercial manufacturing process is defined during this stage based on knowledge gained through development and scale-up activities.

Stage 2 – Process Qualification: During this stage, the process design is evaluated to determine if the process is capable of reproducible commercial manufacturing.

Stage 3 – Continued Process Verification: Ongoing assurance is gained during routine production that the process remains in a state of control.

Types of Process Validation

1. **Prospective Validation:** It is establishment of documented evidence of what a system does or what it purports to do based upon a plan. This validation is conducted prior to the distribution of new product.

2. **Retrospective Validation:** It is the establishment of documented evidence of what a system does or what it purports to do based upon the review and analysis of the existing information. This is conducted in a product already distributed based on accumulated data of production, testing and control.

3. **Concurrent Validation:** It is establishment of documented evidence of what a system does or what it purports to do information generated during implemented of the system.

4. **Revalidation:** Whenever there are changes in packaging, formulation, equipment or processes which could have impact on product effectiveness or product characteristics, there should be revalidation of the validated process.

Conditions that require revalidation studies are:

(a) Changes in critical component

(b) Change in facility or plant

(c) Increase or decrease in batch size

(d) Sequential batches that fail to conform product and process specifications

Change Control: Change control is defined as "a formal system by which qualified representatives of appropriate disciplines review proposed or actual changes that might affect a validated status. The intent is to determine the need for action that would ensure and document that the system is maintained in a validated state."

Change control is a lifetime monitoring approach. Planning for well executed change control procedures includes the following aspects:

Validation Master Plan: It is important to draw up a summarized document that describes the whole project. It has become common practice in the industry to develop a "Validation Master Plan" (VMP). This document would usually include the qualification aspects of a project.

Validation Protocol: After preparing VMP, the next step is to prepare validation protocol. There are the following contents in a validation protocol.

1. General information
2. Objective
3. Background/Prevalidation Activities Summary of development and tech transfer (from R&D or another site) activities to justify in-process testing and controls; any previous validations.
4. List of equipment and their qualification status
5. Facilities qualification
6. Process flow chart
7. Manufacturing procedure narrative
8. List of critical processing parameters and critical excipients
9. Sampling, tests and specifications
10. Acceptance criteria

Process Overview of Tablet Manufacturing

Process step, typical variables and responses during process validation of tablet manufacturing process.

Prospective validation

It is defined as the established documented evidence that a system does what it purports to do based on a preplanned protocol. This validation usually carried out prior to distribution either of a new product or a product made under a revised manufacturing process. Performed on at least three successive production-sizes (Consecutive batches).

In Prospective Validation, the validation protocol is executed before the process is put into commercial use. During the product development phase, the production process should be categorized into individual steps.

Each step should be evaluated on the basis of experience or theoretical considerations to determine the critical parameters that may affect the quality of the finished product. A series of experiment should be designed to determine the criticality of these factors.

Each experiment should be planned and documented fully in an authorized protocol. All equipment, production environment and the analytical testing methods to be used should have been fully validated. Master batch documents can be prepared only after the critical parameters of the process have been identified and machine settings, component specifications and environmental conditions have been determined.

Using this defined process a series of batches should be produced. In theory, the number of process runs carried out and observations made should be sufficient to allow the normal extent of variation and trends to be established to provide sufficient data for evaluation. It is generally considered acceptable that three consecutive batches/runs within the finally agreed parameters, giving product of the desired quality would constitute a proper validation of the process.

In practice, it may take some considerable time to accumulate these data. Some considerations should be exercised when selecting the process validation strategy. Amongst these should be the use of different lots of active raw materials and major excipients, batches produced on different shifts, the use of different equipment and facilities dedicated for commercial production, operating range of the critical processes, and a thorough analysis of the process data in case of Requalification and Revalidation.

During the processing of the validation batches, extensive sampling and testing should be performed on the product at various stages, and should be documented comprehensively. Detailed testing should also be done on the final product in its package.

Upon completion of the review, recommendations should be made on the extent of monitoring and the inprocess controls necessary for routine production.

These should be incorporated into the Batch manufacturing and packaging record or into appropriate standard operating procedures. Limits, frequencies and action to be taken in the event of the limits being exceeded should be specified. Prospective validation should include, but not be limited to the following:

- Short description of the process.
- Summary of the critical processing steps to be investigated.
- List of the equipment/facilities to be used (including measuring, monitoring/recording equipment) together with its calibration status.
- Finished product specifications for release.
- List of analytical methods, as appropriate.
- Proposed in-process controls with acceptance criteria.
- Additional testing to be carried out, with acceptance criteria and analytical validation, as appropriate.
- Sampling plan.
- Methods for recording and evaluating results.
- Functions and responsibilities.
- Proposed timetable

Batches made for process validation should be the same size as the intended Industrial scale batches. If it is intended that validation batches be sold or supplied, the conditions under which they are produced should comply fully with the requirements of Good Manufacturing Practice, including the satisfactory outcome of the validation exercise and the marketing authorization

Concurrent Validation

- It is similar to prospective, except the operating firm will sell the product during the qualification runs, to the public at its market price, and also similar to retrospective validation.

- This validation involves in-process monitoring of critical processing steps and product testing. This helps to generate and documented evidence to show that the production process is in a state of control.

- In exceptional circumstances it may be acceptable not to complete a validation programme before routine production starts.

- The decision to carry out concurrent validation must be justified, documented and approved by authorized personnel.

- Documentation requirements for concurrent validation are the same as specified for prospective validation.

Retrospective Validation

It is defined as the established documented evidence that a system does what it purports to do on the review and analysis of historical information. This is achieved by the review of the historical manufacturing testing data to prove that the process has always remained in control.

This type of validation of a process for a product already in distribution. Retrospective validation is only acceptable for well established processes and will be inappropriate where there have been recent changes in the composition of the product, operating procedures or equipment. Validation of such processes should be based on historical data.

The steps involved require the preparation of a specific protocol and the reporting of the results of the data review, leading to a conclusion and a recommendation.

The source of data for this validation should include, but not be limited to batch processing and packaging records, process control charts, maintenance logbooks, records of personnel changes, process capability studies, finished product data, including trend cards and storage stability results.

Batches selected for retrospective validation should be representative of all batches made during the review period, including any batches that failed to meet the specifications, and should be sufficient in number to demonstrate process consistency.

Additional testing of retained samples may be needed to obtain the necessary amount or type of data to retrospectively validate the process.

For retrospective validation, generally data from ten to thirty consecutive batches should be examined to access process consistency, but fewer batches may be examined if justified.

Some of the essential elements for Retrospective Validation Batches manufactured for a defined period (minimum of 10 last consecutive batches). Number of lots released per year.

- Batch size/strength/manufacturer/year/period.

- Master manufacturing/packaging documents.

- Current specifications for active materials/finished products.

- List of process deviations, corrective actions and changes to manufacturing documents.

- Data for stability testing for several batches.

Revalidation

Re-validation provides the evidence that changes in a process and/or the process environment that are introduced do not adversely affect process characteristics and product quality.

Documentation requirements will be the same as for the initial validation of the process. Facilities, systems, equipment and processes, including cleaning, should be periodically evaluated to confirm that they remain valid.

Where no significant changes have been made to the validated status, a review with evidence that facilities, systems, equipment and processes meet the prescribed requirements fulfils the need for revalidation.

Revalidation becomes necessary in certain situations. Some of the changes that require validation are as follows:

- Changes in raw materials (physical properties such as density, viscosity, particle size distribution and moisture etc that may affect the process or product).

- Changes in the source of active raw material manufacturer.

- Changes in packaging material (primary container/closure system)

- Changes in the process (e.g., mixing time, drying temperatures and batch size)

- Changes in the equipment (e.g., addition of automatic detection system). Changes of equipment which involve the replacement of equipment on a "like for like" basis would not normally require revalidation except that this new equipment must be qualified.

- Changes in the plant/facility. A decision not to perform revalidation studies must be fully justified and documented.

Basic Concept of Process Validation Pharmaceutical Process Validation is the most important and recognized parameters of cGMPs. The requirement of process validation appears of the quality system (QS) regulation. The goal of a quality system is to consistently produce products that are fit for their intended use. Process validation is a key element in assuring that these principles and goal are met. The process validation is standardization of the validation documents that must be submitted with the submission file for marketing authorization. The process validation is intended to assist manufacturers in understanding quality management system (QMS) requirements concerning process validation and has general applicability to manufacturing process.

According to FDA, Assurance of product quality is derived from careful and systemic attention to a number of importance factors, including: selection of quality process through in-process and end product testing. The basic principle for validation may be stated as follows:

Installation Qualification (IQ)

Establishing by objective evidence that all key aspects of the process equipment and ancillary system installation adhere to the manufacturer's approved specification and that the recommendation of the supplier of the equipment are suitably considered. IQ considerations are:

- Equipment design features (i.e. material of construction clean ability, etc.)
- Installation conditions (wiring, utility, functionality, etc.)
- Calibration, preventative maintenance, cleaning schedules.
- Safety features
- Supplier documentation, prints, drawings and manuals.
- Software documented.
- Spare parts list.
- Environmental conditions (such as clean room requirements, temperature, and humidity).

Operational Qualification (OQ)

Establishing by objective evidence process control limits and action levels which result in product that all predetermined requirements.

OQ considerations include:

- Process control limits (time, temperature, pressure, line speed, setup conditions, etc.)
- Software parameters.
- Raw material specifications
- Process operating procedures.

- Material handling requirements.
- Process change control.
- Training.
- Short term stability and capability of the process, (latitude studies or control charts).
- Potential failure modes, action levels and worst-case conditions.
- The use of statistically valid techniques such as screening experiments to optimize the process can be used during this phase.

Performance Qualification (PQ)

- Establishing by objective evidence that the process, under anticipated conditions, consistently produces a product which meets all predetermined requirements. PQ considerations include:
- Actual product and process parameters and procedures established in OQ.
- Acceptability of the product.
- Assurance of process capability as established in OQ.
- Process repeatability, long term process stability.

Re – Qualification Modification to, or relocation of equipment should follow satisfactory review and authorization of the documented change proposal through the change control procedure. This formal review should include consideration of re qualification of the equipment.

Minor changes or changes having no direct impact on final or in-process product quality should be handled through the documentation system of the preventive maintenance program.

The Regulatory Basis for Process Validation

The concept of process validation from its beginnings in the early 1970s through the regulatory aspects associated with current good manufacturing practice (cGMP) regulations and the application thereof to various analytical, quality assurance, pilot plant, production, and sterile product and solid dosage forms considerations.

In the early 1990s, the concept of preapproval inspection (PAI) was born and had as one of its basic tenets the assurance that approved validation protocols and schedules were being generated and that comprehensive development, scale-up, and bio batch and commercial batch validation data were required in order to achieve a successful regulatory PAI audit.

There are several important reasons for validating a product and/or process. First, manufacturers are required by law to conform to cGMP regulations. Second, good business dictates that a manufacturer avoids the possibility of rejected or recalled batches. Third, validation helps to ensure product uniformity, reproducibility, and quality.

Although the original focus of validation was directed towards prescription drugs, the FDA Modernization Act of 1997 expanded the agency's authority to inspect establishments manufacturing over-the-counter (OTC) drugs to ensure compliance with cGMP.

Once the concept of being able to predict process performance to meet user requirements evolved, FDA regulatory officials established that there was a legal basis for requiring process validation. The cGMP regulations for finished pharmaceuticals, 21 CFR 210 and 211, were promulgated to enforce the requirements of the act. FDA has the authority and responsibility to inspect and evaluate process validation performed by manufacturers.

The cGMP regulations for validating pharmaceutical (drug) manufacturing require that drug products be produced with a high degree of assurance of meeting all the attributes they are intended to possess (21 CFR 211.100(a) and 211.110(a)).

Once the concept of being able to predict process performance to meet user requirements evolved, FDA regulatory officials established that there was a legal basis for requiring process validation. The ultimate legal authority is Section 501(a) (2) (B) of the FD&C Act, which states that a drug is deemed to be adulterated if the methods used in, or the facilities or controls used for, its manufacture, processing, packing, or holding do not conform to or were not operated or administrated in conformity with cGMP.

Assurance must be given that the drug would meet the requirements of the act as to safety and would have the identity and strength and meet the quality and purity characteristics that it purported or was represented to possess.

That section of the act sets the premise for process validation requirements for both finished pharmaceuticals and active pharmaceutical ingredients, because active pharmaceutical ingredients are also deemed to be drugs under the act.

The cGMP regulations for finished pharmaceuticals, 21 CFR 210 and 211, were promulgated to enforce the requirements of the act. Although these regulations do not include a definition for process validation, the requirement is implicit in the language of 21 CFR 211.100, which states: "There shall be written procedures for production and process control designed to assure that the drug products have the identity, strength, quality, and purity they purport or are represented to possess." Prerequisite of Process Validation

- Process Development Designee shall review the product development report, data from pilot scale, scale up batch and proposed master formula document of product intended for manufacturing.

- Process Development Designee shall review/ensure the availability analytical method transfer report to the plant and plant preparedness for conducting validation testing and routine testing; function shall co-ordinate with QC/QA in this regards.

- Process Development Designee shall prepare commercial/exhibit batch production and control records which include the operational limits and overall strategy for process control based on development report.

- The Process Validation is performed after the facility, utility, and equipment, and laboratory test methods have been validated and released fir process validation activities. Where compendia method is used only limited analytical method validation shall be conducted.

- All raw material and packaging material specification shall be from approved vendors and shall be approved by quality control.

- All the equipment and instrument to be utilized are calibrated and preventive maintenance programs are in place.

- Relevant SOPs are in place and training is completed on equipment, operation, manufacturing instruction and sampling strategy.

- Key process steps and process variables are identified and their operating ranges have been established.

- All the master formula, manufacturing instruction, packaging instruction, testing procedure and specification shall be approved before execution of process validation batches.

- The cleaning of the area and equipment has been completed prior to the initiation of process validation.

- The validation team and operational team shall be trained from process engineer.

Strategy for Industrial Process Validation of Solid Dosage Forms

- The strategy selected for process validation should be simple and straight-forward. The following five points gives strategy for process validation.

- The use of different lots of raw materials should be included. i.e., active drug substance and major excipients.

- Batches should be run in succession and on different days and shifts (the latter condition, if appropriate).

- Batches should be manufactured in the equipment and facilities designated for eventual commercial production.

- Critical process variables should be set within their operating ranges and should not exceed their upper and lower control limits during process operation. Output responses should be well within finished product specifications.

- Failure to meet the requirements of the Validation protocol with respect to process input and output control should be subjected to process requalification and subsequent revalidation.

Process Validation within the Quality Management System

Process validation is part of the integrated requirements of a quality management system. It is conducted in the context of a system including design and development control, quality assurance, process control, and corrective and preventive action.

The product should be design robustly enough to withstand variations in the manufacturing process and the manufacturing process should be capable and stable to assure continued safe products that perform adequately.

Corrective actions often identify inadequate processes/process validations. Each corrective action applied to a manufacturing process should include the consideration for conducting process validation/ revalidation.

Reason for Process Validation

The possible reason of performing process validation may include:

- New product or existing products as per SUPAC changes.
- Change in site of manufacturing.
- Change in batch size.
- Change in equipment.
- Change in process existing products.
- Change in composition or components.
- Change in the critical control parameters.
- Change in vendor of API or critical excipient.
- Change in specification on input material.
- Abnormal trends in quality parameters of product through review during Annual Product Review (APR).
- Trend of Out of Specification (OOS) or Out of Trend (OOT) in consecutive batches. Benefits of Process Validation
- Consistent through output.
- Reduction in rejections and reworks.
- Reduction in utility cost.
- Avoidance of capital expenditures.
- Fewer complaints about process related failure.
- Reduced testing in process and finished goods.

- More rapid and accurate investigations into process deviation.
- More rapid and reliable start-up of new equipment.
- Easier scale-up from development work.
- Easier maintenance of equipment.
- Improve employee awareness of processes.
- More rapid automation.

Stages of Process Validation

Process Validation is defined as the collection and evaluation of data, from the process design stage through commercial production, which establishes scientific evidence that a process is capable of consistently delivering quality product.

Process Validation involves a series of activities taking place over the lifecycle of the product and process. The activities relating to validation studies may be classified into three stages:

Stage 1 – Process Design

"Focusing exclusively on qualification efforts without also understanding the manufacturing process is defined during this stage based on knowledge gained through development and scale-up activities.

It covers all activities relating to product research and development, formulation, pilot batch studies, scale-up studies, transfer of technology to commercial scale batches, establishing stability conditions, storage and handling of in-process and finished dosage forms, equipment qualification, installation qualification, master production documents, operational qualification, process capability.

Also this is the stage in which the establishment of a strategy for process control is taking place using accumulation knowledge and understanding of the process.

Stage 2 – Process Qualification

During this stage, the process design is evaluated to determine if the process is capable of reproducible commercial manufacturing. It confirms that all established limits of the Critical Process Parameters are valid and that satisfactory products can be produced even under "worst case" conditions. GMP compliant procedures must be followed in this stage and successful completion of this stage is necessary before commercial distribution of a product.

There are two aspect of Process Qualification:

- Design of Facilities and Qualification of Equipment and Utilities : Proper design of manufacturing facility is desired under 21 CFR part 211, subpart

C, of the cGMP regulation on Buildings and Facilities. Activities performed to assure proper facility design and that the equipment and utilities are suitable for their intended use and perform properly.

- Process Performance Qualification "Criteria and process performance indicators that allow for a science and risk-based decision about the ability of the process to consistently produce quality products".

Part of the planning for stage 2 involves defining performance criteria and deciding what data to collect when, how much data, and appropriate analysis of the data. Likely consist of planned comparisons and evaluations of some combination of process measures as well as in-process and trial product attributes. Manufacturer must scientifically determine suitable criteria and justify it. Objective measures, where possible. May be possible to leverage earlier study data if relevant to the commercial scale.

Stage 3 – Continued Process Verification

Ongoing assurance is gained during routine production that the process remains in a state of control. The validation maintenance stage requires frequent review of all process related documents, including validation audit reports to assure that there have been no changes, deviations, failures, modifications to the production process, and that all SOPs have been followed, including change control procedures.

A successful validation program depends on the knowledge and understanding and the approach to control manufacturing processes. These include the source of variation, the limitation of the detection of the variation, and the attributes susceptible of the variation.

For existing products it shall be performed based on matrix approach w.r.t pocket size for blister /strip and different size of HDPE bottles/containers. The activity starts with documenting the change part number and establishing the proven acceptance range

PAR for the machine set parameters e.g.: Sealing temp/speed in blister and strip packing machine, for dry syrups /sterile products speed and sealing torque, for tablets capsules bulk packed in HDPE bottles ,the speed and induction sealing ,power voltage and conveyer speed for topically filled in collapsible tubes ,speed and crimping quality PAR shall be established for each configuration.

Phases in Process Validation

The activities relating to validation studies may be classified into three:

Phase 1: Pre-Validation Qualification Phase

PROCESS DESIGN

Stage 1- PROCESS QUALIFICATION

Stage 2 -CONTINUED PROCESS VERIFICATION

Stage 3 -VALIDATION MAINTENANCE PHASE

Phase 1: Process Qualification

This phase is covers all activities relating to product research and development, formulation pilot batch studies, scale-up studies, transfer of technology to commercial scale batches, establishing stability conditions and storage, and handling of in-process and finished dosage forms, equipment qualification, installation qualification master production document, operational qualification and process capacity.

Phase 2: Process Validation Phase

It is designed to verify that all established limits of the critical process parameter are valid and that satisfactory. Products can be produced even under the worst conditions.

Phase 3: It requires frequent review of all process related documents, including validation of audit reports, to assure that there have been no changes, deviations failures and modifications to the production process and that all standard operating procedures (SOPs), including change control procedures, have been followed. At this stage, the validation team comprising of individuals representing all major departments also assures that there have been no changes/deviations that should have resulted in requalification and revalidation. A careful design and validation of systems and process controls can establish a high degree of confidence that all lots or batches produced will meet their intended specifications. It is assumed that throughout manufacturing and control, operations are conducted in accordance with the principle of good manufacturing practice (GMP) both in general and in specific reference to sterile product manufacture.

Detailed protocols for performing validations are essential to ensure that the process is adequately validated.

Process validation protocols should include the following elements:

- Objectives, scope of coverage of the validation study.
- Validation team membership, their qualifications and responsibilities.
- Type of validation: prospective, concurrent, retrospective, re-validation.
- Number and selection of batches to be on the validation study.
- A list of all equipment to be used; their normal and worst case operating parameters.
- Outcome of IQ, OQ for critical equipment.
- Requirements for calibration of all measuring devices.
- Critical process parameters and their respective tolerances.

- Process variables and attributes with probable risk and prevention shall be captured.
- Description of the processing steps: copy of the master documents for the product.
- Sampling points, stages of sampling, methods of sampling, sampling plans
- Statistical tools to be used in the analysis of data.
- Training requirements for the processing operators.
- Validated test methods to be used in in process testing and for the finished product.
- Specifications for raw and packaging materials and test methods.
- Forms and charts to be used for documenting results.
- Format for presentation of results, documenting conclusions and for approval of study results.

Validation Master Plan

The validation master plan should provide an overview of the entire validation operation, its organizational structure, its content and planning. The main elements of it being the list/inventory of the items to be validated and the planning schedule.

All validation activities relating to critical technical operations, relevant to product and process controls within a firm should be included in the validation master plan. It should comprise all prospective, concurrent and retrospective validations as well as revalidation.

The Validation Master Plan should be a summary document and should therefore be brief, concise and clear. It should not repeat information documented elsewhere but should refer to existing documents such as policy documents, SOP's and validation protocols and reports.

The format and content should include:

- Introduction: validation policy, scope, location and schedule.
- Organizational structure: personnel responsibilities.
- Plant/process/product description: rational for inclusions or exclusions and extent of validation.
- Specific process considerations that are critical and those requiring extra attention.
- List of products/ processes/ systems to be validated, summarized in a matrix format, validation approach.
- Re-validation activities, actual status and
- Key acceptance criteria.

- Documentation format.
- Reference to the required SOP's.
- Time plans of each validation project and sub-project.

Process Validation and Quality Assurance

The relationship of quality assurance and process validation goes well beyond the responsibility of any quality assurance (QA) function. Nevertheless, it is a fair to say that process validation is a QA tool, because it establishes a quality standard for the specific process.

Quality assurance in pharmaceutical companies embodies the effort to assure that products have the strength, purity, safety and efficacy represented in the company's new drug application (NDA) filings.

Although quality assurance is usually designated as a departmental function, it must also be an integral part of an organization's activities. When process validation becomes a general objective of the technical and operational groups within an organization, it becomes the driving force for quality standards in development work, engineering activities, quality assurance, and production.

The quality assurance associated with the pharmaceutical development effort includes the following general functions:

- To ensure that a valid formulation is designated.
- To qualify the process that will be scaled up to production-size batches.
- To assist the design of the validation protocol
- .To manufacture the bio batches for the clinical program, which will become the object of the FDA's preapproval clearance.

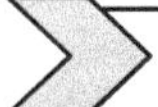 **Conclusion**

Validation is the most widely used word in the areas of drug development, manufacturing and specification of finished products. The consistency and reliability of a validated process to produce a quality product is the very important for an industry. Pharmaceutical Process Validation is the most important and recognized parameters of cGMP. The process validation is intended to assist manufacturers in understanding quality management system (QMS) requirements concerning process validation and has general applicability to manufacturing process. From study, it can be stated that Process validation is a major requirement of cGMP regulation for finished pharmaceutical products. It is a key element in assuring that the quality goals are met. Successfully validating a process may reduce the dependence upon intensive in process and finished product testing. Finally, it can be concluded that Process validation is a key element in the quality assurance of pharmaceutical product as the end product testing is not sufficient to assure quality of finished product.

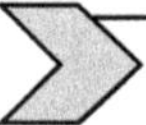 **Important Questions**

1. Who proposed the concept of process validation? Explain in brief?

2. Briefly explain the concept of process validation?

3. It is important to validate a process. Briefly explain this statement?

4. Enlist the elements of validation?

5. What are the different types of process validation?

6. Highlight the importance of Installation qualification, Operational qualification and Performance qualification?

7. What is the strategy for Industrial Process Validation of Solid Dosage Forms?

8. What is Out of specification and Out of trend?

CHAPTER 10

Drug Approval Process in India

The drug approval process in India has faced challenges in recent years, some around compulsory licensing of patents, government price control and narrow standards for patentability. Other issues have also occurred in the clinical trials area, which, despite India's high treatment-naïve population and emerging economy, have reduced pharmaceutical sponsors' interest in India as a priority area in which to conduct clinical studies.

Apart from the CDSCO approval, DCGI has given rights to each state's drug control authority to regulate the manufacture, sale and distribution of drugs. The states include North India: Jammu and Kashmir, Himachal Pradesh, Uttaranchal, Haryana, Panjab; South India: Kerala, Tamilnadu, Karnataka, Andhra Pradesh; East India: West Bengal, Assam, Arunachal Pradesh, Nagaland, Manipur, Mizoram, Tripura, Jharkhand, Bihar, Orrisa; West India: Gujarat, Rajasthan, Maharashtra; and Middle India: Madhya Pradesh, Chhattisgarh. However, final authority does rest with DCGI.

As noted above, challenges emerged between 2011-2013, when the Supreme Court of India had asked for several justifications from the Health Ministry around the conduct and continuance of clinical trials in India after a series of troubling events. The first occurred when a principal investigator was found to have generated fraudulent data and referring patients from a government hospital where he was working, to his private clinic to gain more income.

A regulatory process, by which a person/organization/sponsor/innovator gets authorization to launch a drug or drug product in the market, is known as drug approval process. In general, a drug approval process comprises of various stages: application to conduct clinical trials, conducting clinical trials, application to marketing authorization of drug and post-marketing studies. Every country has its own regulatory authority, which is responsible to enforce the rules and regulations and issue the guidelines to regulate the marketing of the drugs.

SUGAM is e-Governance system to discharge various functions performed by CDSCO under Drugs and Cosmetics Acts, 1940. The software system developed is an online web portal where applicants can apply for NOCs, licenses, registration certificates, permissions & approvals. It provides an online interface for applicants to track their applications, respond to queries and download the permissions issued by CDSCO. It also enables CDSCO officials to process the applications online and generate the permissions online and generate MIS reports.

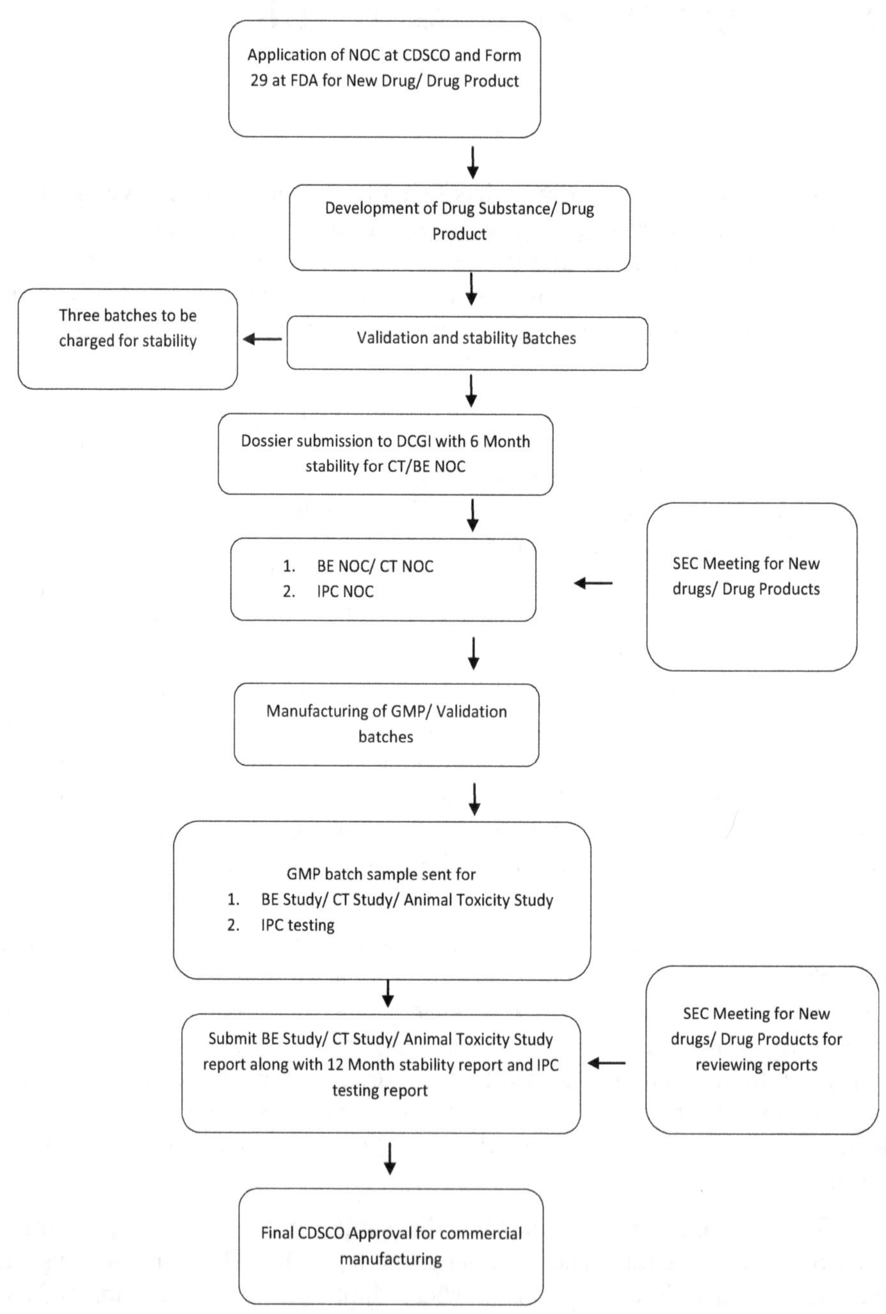

The Health Ministry and stakeholders-including sponsors, CROs, investigators, and the regulatory agency-made a concentrated effort to address the concerns and formed a Subject Experts Committee (SEC, formally known as New Drugs Advisory Committee), Technical Committee and Apex Committee to examine applications for clinical trials in India. All of the studies approved by the DCGI were then evaluated and approved by these committees prior to commencement. Here is a flow chart that demonstrates the process of new product approval in India.

The Health Ministry and stakeholders-including sponsors, CROs, investigators, and the regulatory agency-made a concentrated effort to address the concerns and formed a Subject Experts Committee (SEC, formally known as New Drugs Advisory Committee), Technical Committee and Apex Committee to examine applications for clinical trials in India. All of the studies approved by the DCGI were then evaluated and approved by these committees prior to commencement. Here is a flow chart that demonstrates the process of new product approval in India.

Brief explanation

10.1 Application of Test License (Form-29) at R&D: For any new product first of all No Objection Certificate of **Test License (Form-29)** to be taken from DCGI. For NOC application following documents require for evaluation by drug controller of India and based on documents evaluation, file of **Test License (Form-29)** to be finalised for no objection certificate. Following are the documents list is require for "No Objection Certificate"only for Manufacture Trial and Testing purpose only; and ensure to DCGI that NOC to be used for bioequivalence study as recommended by DCG(I).

Details of documents:
1. Covering letter
2. Affidavit of manufacture
3. API and finished product utilization breakup
4. Finished product specification
5. Finished product slandered testing procedure
6. Specification of Active Pharmaceutical Ingredients (API)
7. Drug license of Active Pharmaceutical Ingredients (API)
8. List of equipment's and instruments with capacity and make details

After receiving the NOC for form 29 application of any new product then form 29 application for research and development to be applied with same documents. We can initiate the any activity related to new product development or any pharmacopoeia listed product in research and development premises after receiving the approved form 29 from CDSCO approval, DCGI has given rights to each state's drug control authority to regulate the guidelines of drugs interim of manufacture, sale and distribution of drugs. The states include North India: Jammu and Kashmir, Himachal Pradesh, Uttaranchal, Haryana, Panjab; South India: Kerala, Tamil Naidu, Karnataka, Andhra Pradesh; East India: West Bengal, Assam, Arunachal Pradesh, Nagaland, Manipur, Mizoram, Tripura, Jharkhand, Bihar, Orrisa; West India: Gujarat, Rajasthan, Maharashtra; and Middle India: Madhya Pradesh, Chhattisgarh. However, final authority does rest with DCGI.

10.2 Development trials at R&D: Once the researcher received the approved Test License (Form-29) from   CDSCO or state's drug control authority which regulate the guidelines of drugs in term of manufacture, sale and distribution of drugs. New product development trails initiate after receiving of approved Test License (Form-29) from CDSCO or state's drug control authority. Active Pharmaceutical Ingredients (API) Procurement, Active Pharmaceutical Ingredients (API) Impurity, Active Pharmaceutical Ingredients (API) Analysis Reagent And Column for analysis to be initiate after receiving of approved Test Licence (Form-29) from CDSCO or state's drug control authority

10.3 New Product Introduction (NPIF): New Product Introduction (NPIF) send to research and development department for information and new product planning by business development team. BD team first evaluate the product market and future forecast of new product based on search of static data and graphical records. Business development team (BDT) also arrange and evaluate the percentage gross cost of any product before finalising the product. Manufacture Company easily predict the future growth of new product in Indian markets based on statics data.

1.4 Technology Transfer of new Product: Technology Transfer of any new product can be initiate after confirmation of the development and analysis of product. When the documents of technology transfer is available, the product development formulation team of plant manufacturing or formulation and research development team will inform to concern department those are directly and indirectly involved in technology transfer of new product as per company standard operation procedures (SOP).

1.5 Three BE batches/EBs to be manufactured at GMP location for stability : As per current DCGI guideline of any dosage form of new product proposal, three exhibit batches or validation batches is mandatory to executed at manufacturing site.

1.6 Dossier filling to DCGI with 6M plant stability data for BE/CT NOC:

The set of documents as per checklist of DCGI dossier to be file along with six month stability data of all condition as per ICH Q1A(R2) Stability Testing of new drugs and products guideline.

Which Content: ICH guidelines regulate the scope necessary for marketing authorization of the stability testing of new active substances and finished medicinal products containing new active substances.) GMP approved manufacturing site **After** receiving NOC from DCGI, BE/CT Study to be performed as per company standard operation procedures (SOP).

1.7 Submission of BE/CT reports and 12M stability data to DCGI for product approval:

The product approval from CDSCO grant is possible only after submitting the following executed plant documents by requested firm.

A) Following list of documents to be require along with validation/Commercial batches for commercial approval :

1. Checklist for Grant of permission to manufacture/import of Bulk Drug already approved in the country S no Documents required to be submitted Enclosed

2. Name of Applicant with address

3. Name of Drug

4. Therapeutic Class

5. Date of Approval

6. Application in Form-44 duly filled and signed by the competent authority

7. Treasury Challan of INR 50,000/- upto 1 year from initial approval and INR 15,000/- for other drugs upto 4 years

7a. For manufacturing:- Copy of manufacturing license in Form-25/ Form-26 for any bulk drug to manufacturer and Form-29

7b. For import:- Copy of drug sale license in Form 20B and 21B

8. Pharmaceutical & Chemical Information

A. Manufacturing Process including flowcharts detailed manufacturing procedure,

i. In process check procedure and report control

ii. Batch manufacturing record

iii. Process validation report.

B. Complete monograph Specifications, methods of analysis including analytical method validation report, with

i. Identification/ quantification of impurities

ii. Enantiomeric purity

iii. Residual solvent/ other volatile impurities (OVI) estimation

C. Structumethodsral elucidation data

D. Three batch Certificate of analysis

E. Stability data of three different lots as per Schedule –Y of Drugs and Cosmetics Rules (should be presented in tabular form with details of Batch no, Batch size, Date of manufacturing, Date of initiation, Packaging details)

F. Material Safety data sheet

G. Reference product characterization

H. Draft specimen Label

9. Sub-acute toxicity data generated with the applicant's bulk drug in two species.

10. CDTL/IPC Test report * * In case of application is for grant of NOC for lab testing serial no 10 may be submitted at the time of approval of bulk drug.

Note: A) Submission requirements / methodology:

(i)   Please submit ONE hard copy and THREE soft copies i.e. Compact Disc (CD) (PDF format, properly bookmarked for navigation) of the dossier.

(ii)   Hard copy: Sides and front of each volume/ file /binder must be labelled with the name of the applicant company, date of submission, name of the drug(s) and the file number (Numbering of files: 'x' of 'y' files e.g. if there are 10 files, file number 6 will be labelled as File No. 6 / 10).

(iii) Use of multiple volumes/ files/ binders is recommended than binding all the documents and modules in a very huge file. Preferably volumes/ files /binders should not be more than 3 inches thick and use of good quality binders is recommended. All the files should be kept together, bound by a good quality wire or thread (If there are too many volumes e.g. more than 10, then multiple grouping should be done).

(iv) CDs have to be labelled using a marker pen with the name of the applicant company, date of submission and name of the drug(s). If there are multiple CDs for one submission dossier, then the numbering as mentioned above should be followed.

(v)   Scanned copies of only signed documents like test reports, signature pages will be acceptable and rest of the document has to be in PDF format with optical character recognition (OCR).

(vi) The table of content under each head should be linked to the files (s) or relevant document for easy tracking in CD's.

(vii) Applicant should preserve a duplicate copy of the submitted dossier for any future reference and should be able to submit multiple copies, if required by CDSCO.

B. Approvals of a New drug (Formulation) already approved in the country following documents are required to be submitted for permission to ferm:

1. Application for permission to Manufacture /Import: (Purpose should be mentioned clearly)

2. Name of the applicant and address

3. Name of the New Drug

a. Composition of the New Drug

b. Dosage Form

c. Proposed indication for the New Drug

d. Therapeutic rational for proposed dosage form

4. Details of the approval of the New Drug in the country

a. Approved Dosage Form details in DCGI reference

b. Approved composition Dosage Form details in DCGI reference

c. Approved indication details in DCGI reference

5. Application in Form 44 duly signed and stamped by authorized personal

6. Treasury challan of INR 15,000 New Drug approved in India for more than one year, or ` 50,000 of New Drug is approved for less than one year duly signed and stamped by Bank of Baroda

7. Copy of valid manufacturing license in Form 25/28/26

8. Copy of valid Test license in Form 29

9. Source of bulk drugs along with current regulatory status of the source with copy of Form 46A/45A. (if obtained)

10. Consent letter and copy of manufacturing licence form supplier of bulk drug

11. Information on active ingredients:

a) Brief Chemical & pharmaceutical data

b) API Specification including impurity profile

c) Method of Analysis with analytical method validation report

d) Certificate of Analysis for three batches

12. Data on Formulation

a) Master manufacturing formula

b) Manufacturing Procedure/ Master manufacturing Record

c) Product development report with Excipient compatibility study and force degradation study.

d) Process validation protocol and Report

e) Finished product specification including impurity profile

f) Finished product Method of Analysis

g) Finished product Analytical method validation report

h) Finished product Certificate of Analysis for three batches/ three validation batches

i) In process quality control check specifications

j) Stability study data report as per requirements of schedule Y mentioning batch size. (should be presented in tabular form with details of Batch no, Batch size, Date of manufacturing, Date of initiation, Packaging details)

k) Dissolution Release Profile (in case of oral dosage form)

l) Comparative Dissolution Release Profile with the Approved formulation (in case of oral dosage form)

m) Comparative evaluation with pharmaceutical equivalence with international brand(s) or approved Indian brands, if applicable

n) Copy of proposed Package Insert which should include generic name of all active ingredients; composition; dosage form/s, indications; dose and method of administration; use in special populations; contraindications; warnings; precautions; drug interactions; undesirable effects; overdose; pharmacodynamics and pharmacokinetic properties; incompatibilities; shelf-life; packaging information; storage and handling instructions.

o) Draft specimen of Label and Carton

13. Regulatory status in other countries, as appropriate.

a) Names of the countries where the drug is marketed/approved for proposed Dosage Form / New Route of Administration along with package insert and/or copies of approval in key countries.

b) Names of the countries where the drug is withdrawn, if any, with reasons c) Free sale certificate (FSC) or Certificate of Pharmaceutical Product (COPP), in case of import.

14. Bio Equivalence/Bioavailability study Protocol (As the case may be)

a) BE protocol

b) Study synopsis

c) Undertaking by investigators as per Appendix VII od schedule Y and CV.

d) Inform consent form (with assurance of providing audio video recordings, Address, qualification, occupation, annual income of subjects along with, name and address of

e) nominee. Compensation clause as per Rule 122 DAB

f) Copy of 'Ethics Committee' approval letters along with registration details.

15. Justification on Bio equivalence study waiver, if requested

16. In case of parenteral formulation, Sub-acute toxicity data conducted with the proposed drug formulation.

17. Submit 11 sets of technical literature (whenever applicable) (10 soft copy and one hard copy) for expert opinion. Each attachment shall not be more than 20 MB in size and shall be properly numbered and named reflecting various sections of the application.

Note : A) Submission requirements / methodology

(i)   Please submit ONE hard copy and THREE soft copies i.e. Compact Disc (CD) (PDF format, properly bookmarked for navigation) of the dossier.

(ii)   Hard copy: Sides and front of each volume/ file /binder must be labelled with the name of the applicant company, date of submission, name of the drug(s) and the file number (Numbering of files: 'x' of 'y' files e.g. if there are 10 files, file number 6 will be labelled as File No. 6 / 10).

(iii) Use of multiple volumes/ files/ binders is recommended than binding all the documents and modules in a very huge file. Preferably volumes/ files /binders should not be more than 3 inches thick and use of good quality binders is recommended. All the files should be kept together, bound by a good quality wire or thread (If there are too many volumes e.g. more than 10, then multiple grouping should be done).

(iv)   CDs have to be labelled using a marker pen with the name of the applicant company, date of submission and name of the drug(s). If there are multiple CDs for one submission dossier, then the numbering as mentioned above should be followed.

(v)   Scanned copies of only signed documents like test reports, signature pages will be acceptable and rest of the document has to be in PDF format with optical character recognition (OCR).

(vi)   The table of content under each head should be linked to the files (s) or relevant document for easy tracking in CD's.

(vii)   Applicant should preserve a duplicate copy of the submitted dossier for any future reference and should be able to submit multiple copies, if required by CDSCO.

B) In case the application is for Clinical Trial /Bio equivalence permission:

a. Adequate chemical and pharmaceutical information should be provided to ensure the proper identity, purity, quality & strength of the investigational product, the amount of information needed may vary with the Phase of clinical trials, proposed duration of trials, dosage forms and the amount of information otherwise available.

b. In case of applications for protocol amendments of already approved studies, applicants should submit copy of approval of protocol, amended new protocol, summarized list of all the new changes incorporated along with justification / reasons for the change.

c. Ethics Committee Approval: Ethical approval should be obtained from Ethics Committee located in the same area where the clinical trial site is located.

d. The proposed clinical trial study centres should be geographically distributed in the country and should also include clinical sites which have their own Institutional Ethics Committee.

3. A drug already approved by the Licensing Authority mentioned in Rule 21 proposed to be marketed with new indication: Following list of documents require for approval

1. Application for permission to manufacture /Import/Clinical trial: (Purpose should be mentioned clearly)

2. Name of the applicant with address

3. Name of the New Drug

a. Composition of the New Drug

b. Dosage Form

c. Proposed indication for the New Drug

d. Therapeutic rational for proposed indication

4. Details of the approval of the New Drug in the country

a. Approved Dosage Form

b. Approved composition

c. Approved indication

5. Application in Form 44 duly signed and stamped by authorized personal

6. Treasury Challan of INR 15,000 New Drug approved in India for more than one year, or INR 50,000 of New Drug is approved for less than one year and not submitted challan earlier for the same drug.

7. Copy of valid manufacturing license in Form 25/28/26

8. Copy of valid Test license in form 29

9. In case of new drug, Source of bulk drugs along with current regulatory status of the source with copy of Form 46A/45A. (if obtained)

10 Consent letter and copy of manufacturing licence form supplier of bulk drug

11. Information on active ingredients:

a) Brief Chemical & pharmaceutical data

b) API Specification with impurity profile

c) Method of Analysis with method validation report

d) Certificate of Analysis for three batches

12. Data on Formulation

a) Master manufacturing formula

b) Manufacturing Procedure/ Master manufacturing Record

c) Product development report with Excipient compatibility and forced degradation study

d) Process validation protocol/ Report

e) Finished product specification

f) Finished product Method of Analysis

g) Finished product Analytical method validation report

h) Finished product Certificate of Analysis for three consecutive batches/ three validation batches

i) In process quality control check specifications

j) Stability study data report as per requirements of schedule Y mentioning batch size. (should be presented in tabular form with details of Batch no, Batch size, Date of manufacturing, Date of initiation, Packaging details)

k) Dissolution Release Profile (in case of oral dosage form)

l) Comparative Dissolution Release Profile with the Approved formulation (in case of oral dosage form)

m) Comparative evaluation with pharmaceutical equivalence with international brand(s) or approved Indian brands, if applicable

n) Copy of proposed Package Insert which should include generic name of all active ingredients; composition; dosage form/s, indications; dose and method of administration; use in special populations; contraindications; warnings; precautions; drug interactions; undesirable effects; overdose; pharmacodynamics and pharmacokinetic properties; incompatibilities; shelf-life; packaging information; storage and handling instructions.

o) Draft specimen of Label and Carton Sr No 10 to 12 is not applicable, if applicant holds manufacturing or Import and marketing permission for the proposed drug product [Except 11(n) and 11(o)]

13. Therapeutic Rationale and justification for the proposed Additional Indication

14. Regulatory status in other countries, as appropriate. a) Names of the countries where the drug is Marketed/ approved for proposed indication along with package insert and/or copies of approval in key countries. b) Names of the countries where the drug is withdrawn, if any, with reasons c) Free sale certificate (FSC) or Certificate of Pharmaceutical Product (COPP), in case of import.

15. Bio Equivalence/Bioavailability study Protocol (As the case may be)

a) BE protocol

b) Study synopsis

c) Undertaking by investigators as per Appendix VII od schedule Y and CV.

d) Inform consent form (with assurance of providing audio-video recordings, Address, qualification, occupation, annual income of subjects along with, name and address of nominee.

e) Compensation clause as per Rule 122 DAB

f) Copy of 'Ethics Committee' approval letters along with registration details.

16. Clinical trial protocol in case of proposed Additional dosage form is not approved in key countries. (Checklist already given in New Drug application)

 I. CT protocol

II. Study synopsis

III. Undertaking by investigators as per Appendix VII of schedule Y and CV.

IV. Inform consent form (with assurance of providing audio-video recordings, Address, qualification, occupation, annual income of subjects along with, name and address of nominee.

V. Compensation clause as per Rule 122 DAB VI. Copy of 'Ethics Committee' approval letters along with registration details.

VII. Case record form (CRF)

VIII. Site details, which includes Investigators name and address, Type of Hospital (Multispecialty/ Government/ Private) , Number of beds, emergency facilities, Ethics Committee registration details, etc)

17. Justification on Clinical trial waiver, if requested.

18. Published report of Clinical trial/Journal/literature with respect to proposed Additional Indication.

19 Submit 11 sets of technical literature (whenever applicable) (10 soft copy and one hard copy) for expert opinion. Each attachment shall not be more than 20 MB in size and shall be properly numbered and named reflecting various sections of the application.

Note: A) Submission requirements / methodology

(i)   One hard copy and three soft copies i.e. Compact Disc (CD) (PDF format) of the dossier.

(ii)   Hard copy: Sides and front of each volume/ file /binder must be labelled with the name of the applicant company, date of submission, name of the drug(s) and the file number (Numbering of files: 'x' of 'y' files e.g. if there are 10 files, file number 6 will be labelled as File No. 6 / 10).

(iii) Use of multiple volumes/ files/ binders is recommended than binding all the documents and modules in a very huge file. Preferably volumes/ files /binders should not be more than 3 inches thick and use of good quality binders is recommended. All the files should be kept together, bound by a good quality wire or thread (If there are too many volumes e.g. more than 10, then multiple grouping should be done).

(iv)   CDs have to be labelled using a marker pen with the name of the applicant company, date of submission and name of the drug(s). If there are multiple CDs for one submission dossier, then the numbering as mentioned above should be followed.

(v)   Scanned copies of only signed documents like test reports, signature pages will be acceptable and rest of the document has to be in PDF format with optical character recognition (OCR).

(vi)   The table of content under each head should be linked to the files (s) or relevant document for easy tracking in CD's. vii. Applicant should preserve a duplicate copy of the submitted dossier for any future reference and should be able to submit multiple copies, if required by CDSCO.

B. In case the application is for clinical trial / Bio equivalence permission:

a. Adequate chemical and pharmaceutical information should be provided to ensure the proper identity, purity, quality & strength of the investigational product, the amount of information needed may vary with the Phase of clinical trials, proposed duration of trials, dosage forms and the amount of information otherwise available.

b. In case of applications for protocol amendments of already approved studies, applicants should submit copy of approval of protocol, amended new protocol, summarized list of all the new changes incorporated along with justification / reasons for the change.

c. Ethics Committee Approval: Ethical approval should be obtained from Ethics Committee located in the same area where the clinical trial site is located.

d. The proposed clinical trial study centres should be geographically distributed in the country and should also include clinical sites which have their own Institutional Ethics Committee.

4. A drug already approved by the Licensing Authority mentioned in Rule 21 and proposed to be marketed as a 'New Dosage Form / New Route of Administration'.

1. Application for permission to Manufacture /Import/Clinical trial: (Purpose should be mentioned clearly)

2. Name of the applicant with address

3. Name of the New Drug

a. Composition of the New Drug

b. Proposed Dosage Form

c. Proposed indication

d. Therapeutic rational for proposed New Dosage Form / New Route

4. Details of the approval of the New Drug in the country

a. Approved Dosage Form and route of administration

b. Approved composition

c. Approved indication

5. Application in Form 44 duly signed and stamped by authorized personal

6. Treasury Challan of INR 15,000 New Drug approved in India for more than one year, or INR 50,000 of New Drug is approved for less than one year and not submitted challan earlier for the same drug.

7. Copy of valid manufacturing license in Form 25/28/26 8. Copy of Test license in form 29

9. In case of new drug, Source of bulk drugs along with current regulatory status of the source with copy of Form 46A/45A. (if obtained)

10. Consent letter and copy of manufacturing licence form supplier of bulk drug

11. Information on active ingredients:

a) Brief Chemical & pharmaceutical data

b) API Specification with impurity profile

c) Method of Analysis with method validation report

d) Certificate of Analysis for three batches

12. Data on Formulation

a) Master manufacturing formula

b) Manufacturing Procedure/ Master manufacturing Record

c) Product development report with Excipient compatibility study and forced degradation study.

d) Process validation protocol/ Report

e) Finished product specification

f) Finished product Method of Analysis

g) Finished product Analytical method validation report

h) Finished product Certificate of Analysis for three consecutive batches/ three validation batches

i) In process quality control check specifications

j) Stability study data report as per requirements of schedule Y mentioning batch size. (should be presented in tabular form with details of Batch no, Batch size, Date of manufacturing, Date of initiation, Packaging details)

k) Dissolution Release Profile (in case of oral dosage form)

l) Comparative Dissolution Release Profile with the Approved formulation (in case of oral dosage form)

m) Comparative evaluation with pharmaceutical equivalence with international brand(s) or approved Indian brands, if applicable

n) Copy of proposed Package Insert which should include generic name of all active ingredients; composition; dosage form/s, indications; dose and method of administration; use in special populations; contraindications; warnings; precautions; drug interactions; undesirable effects; overdose; pharmacodynamic and pharmacokinetic properties; incompatibilities; shelf-life; packaging information; storage and handling instructions.

o) Draft specimen of Label and Carton

13. Therapeutic Rationale and justification for the proposed new dosage form / new route of administration

14. Regulatory status in other countries, as appropriate.

a) Names of the countries where the drug is marketed/approved for proposed Dosage Form / New Route of Administration along with package insert and/or copies of approval in key countries.

b) Names of the countries where the drug is withdrawn, if any, with reasons c) Free sale certificate (FSC) or Certificate of Pharmaceutical Product (COPP), in case of import.

15. Bio Equivalence/Bioavailability study Protocol (As the case may be)

a) BE protocol

b) Study synopsis

c) Undertaking by investigators as per Appendix VII od schedule Y and CV.

d) Inform consent form (with assurance of providing audio-video recordings, Address, qualification, occupation, annual income

e) of subjects along with, name and address of nominee. Compensation clause as per Rule 122 DAB f) Copy of 'Ethics Committee' approval letters along with registration details.

16. Clinical trial protocol in case of proposed Additional dosage form is not approved in key countries. (Checklist already given in New Drug application)

a) CT protocol

b) Study synopsis

c) Undertaking by investigators as per Appendix VII of schedule Y and CV.

d) Inform consent form (with assurance of providing audio-video recordings, Address, qualification, occupation, annual income of subjects along with, name and address of nominee.

e) Compensation clause as per Rule 122 DAB

f) Copy of 'Ethics Committee' approval letters along with registration details.

g) Case record form (CRF)

h) Site details, which includes Investigators name and address, Type of Hospital (Multispecialty/ Government/ Private) , Number of beds, emergency facilities, Ethics Committee registration details, etc)

17. Bio Equivalence study requirement (in case of oral dosage form as appropriate as per Appendix X of Schedule Y)

18. Justification on Clinical trial and Bio equivalence study waiver, if requested.

19. Animal toxicology data as per Schedule Y.

a). Systemic toxicity studies:

i. single dose toxicity

ii. repeated dose toxicity

b). Local toxicity:

i. Dermal toxicity (for products meant for topical (dermal) application)

ii. Ocular toxicity (for products meant for ocular instillation)

iii. Inhalation toxicity (conducted with the formulation proposed to be used via inhalation route)

iv. Vaginal toxicity (for products meant for topical application to vaginal mucosa)

v. Photoallergy or dermal phototoxicity (required if the drug or a metabolite is related to an agent causing photosensitivity or the nature of action suggests such a potential)

c). Rectal tolerance test (For all preparations meant for rectal administration)

20. Published report of Clinical trial/Journal/literature with respect to proposed Dosage Form / New Route of Administration.

21. Submit 11 sets of technical literature (whenever applicable) (10 soft copy and one hard copy) for expert opinion. Each attachment shall not be more than 20 MB in size and shall be properly numbered and named reflecting various sections of the application. Note:

A) Submission requirements / methodology

i. Please submit ONE hard copy and THREE soft copies i.e. Compact Disc (CD) (PDF format) of the dossier.

ii. Hard copy: Sides and front of each volume/ file /binder must be labelled with the name of the applicant company, date of submission, name of the drug(s) and the file number (Numbering of files: 'x' of 'y' files e.g. if there are 10 files, file number 6 will be labelled as File No. 6 / 10).

iii. Use of multiple volumes/ files/ binders is recommended than binding all the documents and modules in a very huge file. Preferably volumes/ files /binders should not be more than 3 inches thick and use of good quality binders is recommended. All the files should be kept together, bound by a good quality wire or thread (If there are too many volumes e.g. more than 10, then multiple grouping should be done).

iv. CDs have to be labelled using a marker pen with the name of the applicant company, date of submission and name of the drug(s). If there are multiple CDs for one submission dossier, then the numbering as mentioned above should be followed.

v. Scanned copies of only signed documents like test reports, signature pages will be acceptable and rest of the document has to be in PDF format with optical character recognition (OCR).

vi. The table of content under each head should be linked to the files (s) or relevant document for easy tracking in CD's.

vii. Applicant should preserve a duplicate copy of the submitted dossier for any future reference and should be able to submit multiple copies, if required by CDSCO.

B. In case the application is for clinical trial / Bio equivalence permission:

a. Adequate chemical and pharmaceutical information should be provided to ensure the proper identity, purity, quality & strength of the investigational product, the amount of information needed may vary with the Phase of clinical trials, proposed duration of trials, dosage forms and the amount of information otherwise available.

b. In case of applications for protocol amendments of already approved studies, applicants should submit copy of approval of protocol, amended new protocol, summarized list of all the new changes incorporated along with justification / reasons for the change.

c. Ethics Committee Approval: Ethical approval should be obtained from Ethics Committee located in the same area where the clinical trial site is located.

d. The proposed clinical trial study centres should be geographically distributed in the country and should also include clinical sites which have their own Institutional Ethics Committee.

5. A drug already approved by the Licensing Authority mentioned in Rule 21 now proposed to be marketed as a 'Modified release dosage form'.

1. Application for permission to Manufacture /Import/Clinical trial: (Purpose should be mentioned clearly)

2. Name of the applicant with address

3. Name of the New Drug

a. Composition of the New Drug

b. Dosage Form

c. Proposed indication for the New Drug

d. Therapeutic rational for Modified release dosage form

4. Details of the approval of the New Drug in the country

 a. Approved Dosage Form and route of administration

b. Approved composition

c. Approved indication

5. Application in Form 44 duly signed and stamped by authorized personal

6. Treasury Challan of INR 15,000 New Drug approved in India for more than one year, or INR 50,000 of New Drug is approved for less than one year and not submitted challan earlier for the same drug.

7. Copy of valid manufacturing license in Form 25/28/26

8. Copy of valid Test license in form 29

9. In case of new drug, Source of bulk drugs along with current regulatory status of the source with copy of Form 46A/45A. (if obtained)

10. Consent letter and copy of manufacturing licence form supplier of bulk drug

11. Information on active ingredients:

a) Brief Chemical & pharmaceutical data

b) API Specification with impurity profiling

c) Method of Analysis with method validation report

d) Certificate of Analysis for three batches

12. Data on Formulation Data on Formulation

a) Master manufacturing formula

b) Manufacturing Procedure/ Master manufacturing Record

c) Product development report with Excipient compatibility study and forced degradation study.

d) Process validation protocol/ Report

e) Finished product specification

f) Finished product Method of Analysis

g) Finished product Analytical method validation report

h) Finished product Certificate of Analysis for three consecutive batches/ three validation batches

i) In process quality control check specification

j) Stability study data report as per requirements of schedule Y mentioning batch size. (should be presented in tabular form with details of Batch no, Batch size, Date of manufacturing, Date of initiation, Packaging details)

k) Dissolution Release Profile (in case of oral dosage form)

l) Comparative Dissolution Release Profile with the Approved formulation (in case of oral dosage form)

m) Comparative evaluation with pharmaceutical equivalence international brand(s) or approved Indian brands, if applicable

n) Copy of proposed Package Insert which should include generic name of all active ingredients; composition; dosage form/s, indications; dose and method of administration; use in special populations; contraindications; warnings; precautions; drug interactions; undesirable effects; overdose; pharmacodynamic and pharmacokinetic properties; incompatibilities; shelf-life; packaging information; storage and handling instructions.

o) Draft specimen of Label and Carton

13. Therapeutic Rationale and justification for the proposed new dosage form / new route of administration

14. Regulatory status in other countries, as appropriate.

a) Names of the countries where the drug is marketed/approved for proposed Modified Dosage Form along with package insert and/or copies of approval in key countries.

b) Names of the countries where the drug is withdrawn, if any, with reasons

c) Free sale certificate (FSC) or Certificate of Pharmaceutical Product (COPP), in case of import.

15. Bio Equivalence/Bioavailability study Protocol (As the case may be)

a) BE protocol

b) Study synopsis

c) Undertaking by investigators as per Appendix VII od schedule Y and CV.

d) Inform consent form (with assurance of providing audio-video recordings, Address, qualification, occupation, annual income

e) of subjects along w Compensation clause as per Rule 122 DAB birth, name and address of nominee.

f) Copy of 'Ethics Committee' approval letters along with registration details.

16. Clinical trial protocol in case of proposed Additional dosage form is not approved in key countries. (Checklist already given in New Drug application)

a) CT protocol

b) Study synopsis

c) Undertaking by investigators as per Appendix VII of schedule Y and CV.

d) Inform consent form (with assurance of providing audiovideo recordings, Address, qualification, occupation, annual income of subjects along with, name and address of nominee.

e) Compensation clause as per Rule 122 DAB

f) Copy of 'Ethics Committee' approval letters along with registration details.

g) Case record form (CRF)

h) Site details, which includes Investigators name and address, Type of Hospital (Multispecialty/ Government/ Private) , Number of beds, emergency facilities, Ethics Committee registration details, etc)

17. Bio Equivalence study requirement (in case of oral dosage form as appropriate as per Appendix X of Schedule Y)

18. Justification on Clinical trial and Bio equivalence study waiver, if requested.

19. Published report of Clinical trial/Journal/ literature with respect to proposed Modified Dosage Form.

20. In case of injectable formulation, sub-acute toxicity data conducted with the applicant drug formulation. 21. Submit 11 sets of technical literature (whenever applicable) (10 soft copy and one hard copy) for expert opinion. Each attachment shall not be more than 20 MB in size and shall be properly numbered and named reflecting various sections of the application.

Note: A) Submission requirements / methodology

i. Firm can submit one hard copy and three soft copies i.e. Compact Disc (CD) (PDF format) of the dossier.

ii. Hard copy: Sides and front of each volume/ file /binder must be labelled with the name of the applicant company, date of submission, name of the drug(s) and the file number (Numbering of files: 'x' of 'y' files e.g. if there are 10 files, file number 6 will be labelled as File No. 6 / 10).

iii. Use of multiple volumes/ files/ binders is recommended than binding all the documents and modules in a very huge file. Preferably volumes/ files /binders should not be more than 3 inches thick and use of good quality binders is recommended. All the files should be kept together, bound by a good quality wire or thread (If there are too many volumes e.g. more than 10, then multiple grouping should be done).

iv. CDs have to be labelled using a marker pen with the name of the applicant company, date of submission and name of the drug(s). If there are multiple CDs for one submission dossier, then the numbering as mentioned above should be followed.

v. Scanned copies of only signed documents like test reports, signature pages will be acceptable and rest of the document has to be in PDF format with optical character recognition (OCR).

vi. The table of content under each head should be linked to the files (s) or relevant document for easy tracking in CD's. vii. Applicant should preserve a duplicate copy of the submitted dossier for any future reference and should be able to submit multiple copies, if required by CDSCO.

B. In case the application is for clinical trial / Bio equivalence permission:

a. Adequate chemical and pharmaceutical information should be provided to ensure the proper identity, purity, quality & strength of the investigational product, the amount of information needed may vary with the Phase of clinical trials, proposed duration of trials, dosage forms and the amount of information otherwise available.

b. In case of applications for protocol amendments of already approved studies, applicants should submit copy of approval of protocol, amended new protocol, summarized list of all the new changes incorporated along with justification / reasons for the change.

c. Ethics Committee Approval: Ethical approval should be obtained from Ethics Committee located in the same area where the clinical trial site is located.

d. The proposed clinical trial study centres should be geographically distributed in the country and should also include clinical sites which have their own Institutional Ethics Committee.

6. A drug already approved by the Licensing Authority mentioned in Rule 21 proposed to be marketed with Additional Strength, list of documents require

1. Application for permission to Manufacture /Import/Clinical trial: (Purpose should be mentioned clearly)

2. Name of the applicant with address

3. Name of the New Drug

a. Composition of the New Drug

b. Dosage Form

c. Proposed indication for the New Drug

4. Details of the approval of the New Drug in the country :

a. Approved Dosage Form

b. Approved composition

c. Approved Strength along with Indication

5. Application in Form 44 duly signed and stamped by authorized personal

6. Treasury Challan of INR 15,000 New Drug approved in India for more than one year, or INR 50,000 of New Drug is approved for less than one year and not submitted challan earlier for the same drug.

7. Copy of valid manufacturing license in Form 25/28/26

8. Copy of Test license in form 29

9. in case of new drug, Source of bulk drugs along with current regulatory status of the source with copy of Form 46A/45A. (If obtained)

10. Consent letter and copy of manufacturing licence form supplier of bulk drug

11. Information on active ingredients:

a) Brief Chemical & pharmaceutical data

b) API Specification with impurity

c) Method of Analysis with method validation report

d) Certificate of Analysis for three batches

12. Data on Formulation

a) Master manufacturing formula

b) Manufacturing Procedure/ Master manufacturing Record

c) Product development report

d) Process validation protocol/ Report with Excipient compatibility study and Forced degradation profile.

e) Finished product specification

f) Finished product Method of Analysis

g) Finished product Analytical method validation report

h) Finished product Certificate of Analysis for three consecutive batches/ three validation batches

i) In process quality control check specification

j) Stability study data evaluation a s per requirements of schedule Y mentioning batch size. . (should be presented in tabular form with details of Batch no, Batch size, Date of manufacturing, Date of initiation, Packaging details)

k) Dissolution Release Profile (in case of oral dosage form)

l) Comparative Dissolution Release Profile with the Approved formulation (In case of oral dosage form)

m) Comparative evaluation with international brand(s) or approved Indian brands, if applicable

n) Copy of proposed Package Insert which should include generic name of all active ingredients; composition; dosage form/s, indications; dose and method of administration; use in special populations; contraindications; warnings; precautions; drug interactions; undesirable effects; overdose; pharmacodynamics and pharmacokinetic properties; incompatibilities; shelf-life; packaging information; storage and handling instructions.

o) Draft specimen of Label and Carton Information on active ingredients:

13. Therapeutic Rationale and justification for the proposed Additional Strength

14. Regulatory status in other countries, as appropriate.

a) Names of the countries where the drug is Marketed/ approved for proposed additional strength along with package insert and/or copies of approval in key countries.

b) Names of the countries where the drug is withdrawn, if any, with reasons

c) Free sale certificate (FSC) or Certificate of Pharmaceutical Product (COPP), in case of import.

15. Bio Equivalence/Bioavailability study Protocol (As the case may be)

a) BE protocol

b) Study synopsis

c) Undertaking by investigators as per Appendix VII od schedule Y and CV.

d) Inform consent form (with assurance of providing audio-video recordings, Address, qualification, occupation, annual income

e) of subjects along with, name and address of nominee. Compensation clause as per Rule 122 DAB

f) Copy of 'Ethics Committee' approval letters along with registration details.

16. Clinical trial protocol in case of proposed Additional Strength is not approved in key countries. (Checklist already given in New Drug application)

a. CT protocol

b. Study synopsis

c. Undertaking by investigators as per Appendix VII of schedule Y and CV.

d. Inform consent form (with assurance of providing audio-video recordings, Address, qualification, occupation, annual income of subjects along with, name and address of nominee.

e. Compensation clause as per Rule 122 DAB

f. Copy of 'Ethics Committee' approval letters along with registration details.

g. Case record form (CRF)

h. Site details, which includes Investigators name and address, Type of Hospital (Multispecialty/ Government/ Private) , Number of beds, emergency facilities, Ethics Committee registration details, etc)

17. Justification on Clinical trial and Bio equivalence study waiver, if requested.

18. Published report of Clinical trial/Journal/literature with respect to proposed Additional Strength.

19. In case of injectable formulation, sub-acute toxicity data conducted with the applicant drug formulation. 20. Submit 11 sets of technical literature (whenever applicable) (10 soft copy and one hard copy) for expert opinion. Each attachment shall not be more than 20 MB in size and shall be properly numbered and named reflecting various sections of the application.

Note: A) Submission requirements / methodology

i.   Please submit ONE hard copy and THREE soft copies i.e. Compact Disc (CD) (PDF format) of the dossier.

ii.   Hard copy: Sides and front of each volume/ file /binder must be labelled with the name of the applicant company, date of submission, name of the drug(s) and the file number (Numbering of files: 'x' of 'y' files e.g. if there are 10 files, file number 6 will be labelled as File No. 6 / 10).

iii. Use of multiple volumes/ files/ binders is recommended than binding all the documents and modules in a very huge file. Preferably volumes/ files /binders should not be more than 3 inches thick and use of good quality binders is recommended. All the files should be kept together, bound by a good quality wire or thread (If there are too many volumes e.g. more than 10, then multiple grouping should be done).

iv.   CDs have to be labelled using a marker pen with the name of the applicant company, date of submission and name of the drug(s). If there are multiple CDs for one submission dossier, then the numbering as mentioned above should be followed.

v.   Scanned copies of only signed documents like test reports, signature pages will be acceptable and rest of the document has to be in PDF format with optical character recognition (OCR).

vi.   The table of content under each head should be linked to the files (s) or relevant document for easy tracking in CD's.

vii. Applicant should preserve a duplicate copy of the submitted dossier for any future reference and should be able to submit multiple copies, if required by CDSCO.

B. In case the application is for clinical trial / Bio equivalence permission:

a. Adequate chemical and pharmaceutical information should be provided to ensure the proper identity, purity, quality & strength of the investigational product, the amount of information needed may vary with the Phase of clinical trials, proposed duration of trials, dosage forms and the amount of information otherwise available.

b. In case of applications for protocol amendments of already approved studies, applicants should submit copy of approval of protocol, amended new protocol, summarized list of all the new changes incorporated along with justification / reasons for the change.

c. Ethics Committee Approval: Ethical approval should be obtained from Ethics Committee located in the same area where the clinical trial site is located.

d. The proposed clinical trial study centres should be geographically distributed in the country and should also include clinical sites which have their own Institutional Ethics Committee.

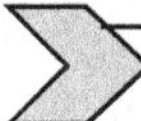 **Important Questions**

1. What is the difference between DCGI and CDSCO?

2. What are the functions of DCGI?

3. What is Form 29?

4. What is import licensee and test Licence?

5. Define the CT 11 NOC and list of documents require for application of the same.

6. Define the rules of BE NOC as per CDSCO Instruction.

7. What are the list of documents require for dossier filing in CDSCO?

8. What Form is required before introducing a new product in R&D? Explain in brief.

9. Briefly explain the Complete DCGI filing process.

CHAPTER 11

Regulatory Requirements for Dossier Filing in ROW and International Markets

A new molecule can cost several millions of rupees or dollars to progress and any blunder causes greater impact on company's status. As medicines play a vital role in human's life there must be regulations for medicines ensuring Quality, Safety and Efficacy of drugs. The regulatory affairs professional is the only one who is completely responsible for holding products in compliance and maintaining all the records. One of the vital activities of the regulatory specialist is to ensure that the all the information regarding medicines has been correctly established to the patient covering labeling also.

Even a small mistake in any of the activities related to regulatory can make the product to be recall in addition to loss of several millions of the money. The current Pharmaceutical Industry is well organized, systematic and compliant to international regulatory standards for manufacturing of Chemical and Biological drugs for human and veterinary consumption as well as medical devices, traditional herbal products and cosmetics. Drug development to materialistically is highly controlled.

Every drug before acquire market approval must undergo meticulous inspection and clinical trials to make sure its safety, efficacy and quality. These standards are brought by regulatory authorities of their corresponding countries like as FDA in US and DCA in India etc. Regulation influences all strands of the pharmaceutical world, from maverick pioneers and pharmaceutical companies to regulatory and managerial bodies and patients also.

Regulatory department is pivotal interface between company, products and regulatory authorities whose positive or negative vantage point to strengthen the discernment of the regulatory authority into the industry, for good or for bad. So, the better the scientific exactitude, the greater will be the chances for a product to come to the market within the expected time.

Evolution of regulatory affairs

In 1950's generation, many tragedies came about due to the misinterpretation of the employees during manufacture & some purposive addition of contaminated substances into the pharmaceutical product which has move forward to the execution of the patients. After so many occurrences, the regulatory bodies launched the new laws and guidelines which are going to ameliorate the quality, safety and efficacy of the products. This is again developed into severe standards for Marketing Authorization (MA) and Good Manufacturing Practices (GMPs). That is the tragedies of SULPHANILAMIDE ELIXIR, VACCINE TRAGEDY & THALIDOMIDE TRAGEDY.

FDA launched in 1906 as Bureau of chemistry, served simply to police claims made about food and drugs ingredients. At that time no formal government approval required to market new drugs. The disasters provoked a public outcry that led to the passage of the 1983 Food Drug & Cosmetics Act, which gave the FDA power to monitor the safety of new drug.

Scope of regulatory affairs in pharmaceutical industry

The regulation of medical products has been expanding since early 20th century. Regulatory agencies are being established in an ever increasing number of countries across the globe. Those that have established are reorganizing their systems and attempting to harmonize with organizations of other countries.

The pharmaceutical, biotechnology and medical devices are among the most highly regulated industries in the world. Regulatory affairs (RA) professionals are employed in pharmaceutical industry, government, academic research and clinical institutions. The Indian Pharmaceutical industry is one of the fastest growing industries in India, with a compounded annual growth rate (CAGR) of over 13 % in last 5 years and it is expected to grow at a higher rate in coming 10 years. It is valued at $ 8.0 billion approximately and ranks 4th in terms of volume and 13th in terms of value globally. All companies engaged in R&D worth its salt has an individual RA department to aid them in new product development. The clinical research industry, which provides opportunities for RA professionals, is also growing at an unparalleled rate. It has opened up new vistas of employment for a large number of trained professionals. The clinical trials market worldwide is worth over USD 52 billion. A study by Ernst and Young indicates that the total market value of Clinical Research activities performed in India is expected to grow to around USD 1.5-2 billion. There is expected to be a huge demand for qualified RA personnel in clinical research.

"Diseases that cannot be cured, diseases that have to be managed, provide great opportunities for generic drugs." Government has the responsibility to protect their citizens. It is the responsibility of national governments to establish regulatory authorities with strong guidelines for quality assurance and drug regulations in the respective territories.

Somewhat parallel with the ongoing harmonization and movement toward creating a common market for medicines inside the EU, the need for wider harmonization was felt by officials from Japan, EU, and US during International Conference of Drug Regulatory Authorities (ICDRA) organized by world health organization (WHO).

The informal discussions had led to a need of the harmonization of requirements relating to the new innovative drugs and also subsequently paved the way to the establishment of International Conference on Harmonization of Technical Requirements for the Registration of Pharmaceuticals for Human Use (ICH), a collaborative initiative between the EU, Japan, and the United States with observers from WHO, EFTA, and Canada. Efforts to harmonize various elements of drug regulatory activities have been initiated by various inter-governmental organizations at regional and interregional level in the past decade. The driving force behind these efforts has been the increase in global trade in pharmaceutical products, and growth in the complexity of technical regulations related to drug efficacy, safety, and quality.

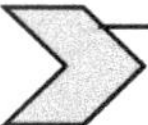 ## Generic Drug Development

To make a generic product, formulator must know in detail the exact regulatory requirements of each concerned country where the drug is intended to be filed. Generic drug product development uses a different approach and strategy compared to that used to develop an innovator drug product containing a new chemical entity.

Generic drug product manufacturers must formulate a drug product that will have the same therapeutic efficacy, safety, and performance characteristics as of its branded counterpart. The key factor is that the generic drug product must meet all the necessary criteria to be therapeutically equivalent to the innovator drug product.

Therapeutically equivalent means that the drug product shows pharmaceutical equivalence as well as bioequivalence. The decision to proceed with the development of a generic drug product should therefore be based on well-researched data that primarily indicate market value together with a sound knowledge of patent expiry dates, predicted market share, and growth rate for the product, amongst others.

The predicted profitability of the new generic product will require strategic planning for the subsequent launch timing, which must take into account the expected generic price and knowledge of anticipated competitors, such as who they are and when they are expected. According to HamrellR.Michael "The Drug Price Competition and Patent Term Restoration Act" in 1984 changed the regulatory climate for generic drugs. This law allowed for the approval of generic "me-too" copies of many approved drug after the patent had expired. As per Kathy Redmond the regulatory agencies have a responsibility to ensure that high-quality, safe, and effective medicines are made available to patients in a timely manner. Despite the fact that all regulators worldwide share the same aims, they do not adopt a consistent approach to drug approval requirements, and as a result, medicines are often approved quicker in some countries than others. Therefore, there is need for a harmonized drug regulation globally.

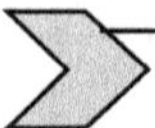

Filing a Generic Drug Application

When a dossier is ready as per the regulatory requirement of the respective country, it is submitted to the regulatory agency of that country. Various regulatory agencies worldwide are tabulated in the Table 2. Food and Drug Administration(FDA), European Medicines Agency (EMA), Pharmaceutical and Medical Devices Agency (PMDA), Therapeutic Goods Administration (TGA), South Africa Health Product Regulatory Authority (SAHPRA), Medicines Control Council (MCC), Tanzania Food and Drugs Authority (TFDA), Agência Nacional De Vigilância Sanitária (National Health Surveillance Agency) (ANVISA), Commonwealth Independent States (CIS), Department of Health (DOH), The Gulf Co-Operation Council (GCC).

United States of America

USA is the major market for the pharmaceutical industry. The USA has evolved from no regulations in the 18th century to one of the highly regulated and admired regulatory authority in the world. The food and drug administration (FDA) within the U.S. Department of Health and Human Services regulates the drug approval system in United States with help of six product centers including Center for Drug Evaluation and Research (CDER).

Drug registration in USA is majorly categorized by two types of applications: New Drug Application (NDA) and Abbreviated New Drug Application (ANDA). ANDA is filled for generic drug products; those require marketing authorization and are of exact or close copies of already approved drugs. The ANDA approval process is depicted in Figure 1[7] Indeed, the way this country regulates drugs typically has been born out of adversity, out of events that have killed and injured thousands.

The evolution of the current drug regulatory system in USA is recognized globally as the gold standard for drug safety and efficacy. During 1990, FDA began work to develop standards for the exchange of electronic information critical to the agency's mission. This recognized both the inefficiency of paper for transferring mass quantities of data and the need to develop a harmonized format that would be usable by FDA as well as its counterparts in the European Union and Japan. Consequently, firms are now able to submit paperless product applications and related material to world regulatory agencies more efficiently, while each review authority maintains its own high standards for product evaluation.

Because all drugs have some risk, FDA task force advised the agency to make more systematic use of the principles of risk management in the way FDA oversees drug development and marketing.

Name of Country/ Group	Regulatory authority
USA	FDA
EU	EMA
Canada	Health Canada
Japan	PMDA
Australia	TGA
South Africa	SAHPRA
AFRICA (Tanzania)	Independent regulatory agencies/TFDA
Brazil	ANVISA
Russia	Federal Agency for Healthcare and Social Development Supervision

European Union

The EU has one of the most highly regarded regulatory systems in the world. The system comprises of European parliament, the council of ministers, and the European Commission. EU consists of 27 member states: Austria, Belgium, Bulgaria, Cyprus, Czech Republic, Denmark, Estonia, Finland, France, Germany, Greece, Hungary, Ireland, Italy, Latvia, Lithuania, Luxemburg, Malta, Netherlands, Poland, Portugal, Romania, Slovakia, Slovenia, Spain, Sweden, and the United Kingdom and three countries which are member of European Free Trade Agreement (EFTA) Iceland, Norway, and Liechtenstein.[8] These EFTA members are those countries which were unable to join rest of the 27 member states as common market. These three EFTA member countries along with 27 EU member states, comprises of the European Economic Area (EEA). The European Medicines Agency is a decentralized agency of the European Union, located in London.[8] The Agency is responsible for the scientific evaluation of medicines developed by pharmaceutical companies for use in the European Union and applications for European marketing authorizations for both human and veterinary medicines (centralized procedure). Under the centralized procedure, companies submit a single marketing-authorization application to the Agency. Once granted by the European Commission, a centralized (or "Community") marketing authorization is valid in all European Union (EU) and EEA-EFTA states (Iceland, Liechtenstein and Norway). The European parliament approves the laws together with the council of ministers. The council of ministers is the voice of Member states and is responsible for enactment of directives.

Types of submission procedure

To market a generic medicinal product in European Economic Area (EEA) which consists of 27 member states and 3 EFTA countries, a marketing authorization has to be issued. European medicines Agency (EMA formerly known as EMEA) regulates the medicinal products marketing authorization through various committees. In case of Generic drug products, generally the decentralized procedure is followed whereas in case of the new drug products the application for marketing authorization is always submitted through a centralized procedure.

Brazil

Brazil's pharmaceutical market is the 11th largest in the world and second in Latin America after Mexico since the devaluation of 2001.Brazil's market is clearly a key market to drive the global development of any pharmaceutical company with international ambitions and may have located regional headquarters in the country. The regulatory framework is considerably improved and makes Brazil a preferred gateway to other Latin American markets. The federal regulatory agency responsible for pharmaceutical product registration in Brazil is ANVISA (National Sanitary Vigilance agency), which was established in 1999. The 1999 Law (The Generics Law) and the ANVISA regulate the implementation of generic pharmaceuticals policy in Brazil, establishes the technical standards and defines the concepts of bioavailability, bioequivalent drugs, innovators, reference drugs, and similar. According to the Brazilian legislation, all the pharmaceutical products must be registered with ANVISA before coming to market in Brazil. Product registration in Brazil is a laborious exercise, and is to be requested by the local Brazilian based office of the foreign company or its distributor in Brazil. The registration is valid for 5 years and can be renewed continuously for the same period. Law must complete the registration process within 90 days after the registration is requested, or denied. For registration purposes, ANVISA classifies the products in various categories. The medications for human use are divided into three distinct areas i.e., New Product, Similar Product, Generic Product

Tanzania (AFRICA)

African medicines regulatory authorities (MRAs) role is to ensure that the pharmaceutical products those are needed, are registered in their country: This process is called "registration," "marketing approval," "marketing authorization" or "product licensing", and involves assessment of product information submitted by the manufacturer (the product 'dossier') to make sure that it is safe and effective for use by local patients. Assessment of generic drugs is relatively simple. This is because the regulator only needs to establish two key points. First, generic drug product is bioequivalent to and thus therapeutically interchangeable with the comparator product. Secondly, product meets comparable sustainable quality standards to that of the innovator product. Every country of the African region has its own regulatory framework. Drug product registration was gradually introduced in Tanzania under the Tanzania Food, Drugs and Cosmetics Act 2003, to have a smooth transition, beginning with 1-year provisional registration taken as a notification from 1998. This gave ample time for the Pharmacy Board to prepare guidelines to assist applicants and evaluators to respectively submit and evaluate correctly the required information. Following the preparation of the guidelines, the first application was received in 1997 and the first product was registered in April 1999.All documents shall be in Kiswahili or English. Applications that do not comply to requirements prescribed in these guidelines will be rejected and returned to the applicant at his own cost. All ingredients used in the formulation of generic medicinal products must comply with specifications prescribed either in the USP (United States pharmacopoeia), BP (British pharmacopoeia), EP (European pharmacopoeia), and International or Japanese pharmacopoeia. In-house specifications shall only be accepted if the limits are tighter than those prescribed in those pharmacopoeias and other specifications may be accepted if they are validated.

Russia

According to some estimates, Russia is poised to be among the top five Global pharmaceutical markets in terms of value in the next five years.[13] Today, Russia stands at the threshold of becoming a major force in the global pharmaccutical markct. Russia is a mcmbcr country of "Thc Commonwcalth of Independent States" (CIS) founded in 1991, which is a regional organization whose participating countries are former Soviet Republics, formed after the dissolution of the Union of Soviet Socialist Republics (USSR). The regulatory processes in CIS countries are led and supervised by Regulatory Agencies closely collaborating with or operating within the respective Ministries of Health. Each of the CIS countries has established individual registration guidelines. Registration in RUSSIA is a national procedure. Estimated duration of procedure is up to 24 months. Documentation is done in Russian language in format compliant with Russian requirements. Recommended submission of a bioequivalence study is carried out in certified research organizations within the Russian Federation's territory. Original and generic products pass the same stages of registration. Original products must pass through all registration procedures while the generic products are exempted from some of them. For example, original product must undergo clinical trials in Russia. For generic products, bio-equivalence studies can be conducted in any other countries and not only in Russia.

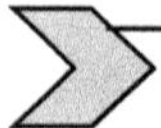 ## Conclusion

Although there is a continuous process of harmonization taking place all around the world, still we see a huge challenge, which is yet to be overcome by the Pharmaceutical industry in case of generic drug development and filing. This is due to the heterogeneity in the regulatory landscape of the various countries. Therefore, to meet these challenges, a lot of strategic planning is required before the development of any generic drug product.

The path a drug travels from a lab to your medicine cabinet is usually long, and every drug takes a unique route. Often, a drug is developed to treat a specific disease. An important use of a drug may also be discovered by accident. Most drugs that undergo preclinical (animal) testing never even make it to human testing and review by the FDA.

The drugs that do must undergo the agency's rigorous evaluation process, which scrutinizes everything about the drug--from the design of clinical trials to the severity of side effects to the conditions under which the drug is manufactured. As noted, the parts played by the FDA and industry are well defined.

A big step is to be an advocate for drug development and stewardship. Providers should ask if the current drug armamentarium for a condition or disease is ideal. Knowing treatment limitations and understanding how care could be optimized with newer drugs, dosages, and delivery routes, while limiting adverse events, are important in advocacy.

Product development is supported by having new clinical sites and working to have diverse study populations. Pediatric infectious diseases providers or institutions that use a product multiple times.

Providers should be open for partaking in studies and could potentially have trainees learn about the process as well. Institutions should also consider establishing provider time support and clinical space for studies. Providers can work with sponsors to understand gaps or limitations that are causing delays in the progression to NDAs; the FDA may be able to advise on combining efforts among institutions or modeling data to help hasten perceived roadblocks. As funding for clinical trials is often lacking, it is important for physicians to work with sponsors to approach the FDA for accelerated approval or orphan drug status for qualifying products, as well as lobbying for legislature, which promotes funding constructs for products. The process of drug development is complex interwoven effort among scientists, patients, industry sponsors, FDA, and prescribing providers, with each group having a critical role to play.

About the Author

Dr. Arun Kumar Pandey

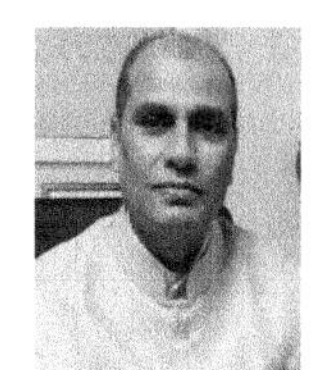

Sr.Vice President (Alkem Laboratories Limited) is a performance-driven humanitarian, academician, researcher and a personality having profound deep-seated knowledge in the domain of research and development. As a mascot, leader and executor, responsible for holding 500 scientists to augment and guide in their work of research, development and formulating innovative products in the domain of the pharmaceutical field, where expertise and prolific knowledge impales and stand out exclusively.

Deftness in developing new formulations, existing processes and their manufacturing, purchase and maintenance-related activities with a chain of managers adept at new technical platforms of innovations with new patent filing, clinical development and strategic planning for execution of technology with an outstanding 'track record' of leading the development and implementation of new procedures.

As an erudite scholar, thinker, innovator and sound administrator has a tangible hold in the realm of man-management and leaves no doubts, for abilities in all these fields ensemble with the understanding of fintech, financial facts and figures and immense problem-solving skills coupled with thinking out of the box ability.

As a scholar and academician par excellence, work and publication have left an indelible impact in national and international journals. The work recently published delves deep into herbal therapy of parasitic infections caused by helminths and is evaluated and published in renowned international journals by "Elsevier Science Direct". "Nanosponges: A recent technology for nanomedicine" published in Pharma Innovation Journal shows interest in the novel drug development.

Innovations related to various national and international patent attorneys are expected to enlighten and enthral the readers. "Oral pharmaceutical compositions of amorphous Apremilast and process for preparing thereof", "Stable pharmaceutical composition of active fragments of basic fibroblast of preparation thereof"; and another patent related to novel drug delivery reflecting the innovative ideas of discovery.

During an illustrious career which has spun over two immemorable decades of scholarly work and service-oriented activities, Efforts has been decorated with myriad, handsome emoluments and epithets which have become the important cornerstone of my career as an organizational coach, mentor, prolific speaker, innovator, an able administrator and an acclaimed scientist and also an impaling researcher who stands out with all exclusivity; and has created an everlasting influence in the realm science and humanity growth factor (Bf gf) for treating vitiligo and process.